Away with all pests

Joshua S. Horn, M.D.

Away with all pests

An English surgeon in People's China:
1954-1969

Introduction by Edgar Snow

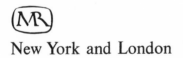

New York and London

Library of Congress Catalog Card Number: 73-142988

First Modern Reader Paperback Edition 1971
20 19 18 17 16 15 14 13 12 11 10

Monthly Review Press
62 West 14th Street, New York, N.Y. 10011
47 Red Lion Street, London WC1R 4PF

Manufactured in the United States of America

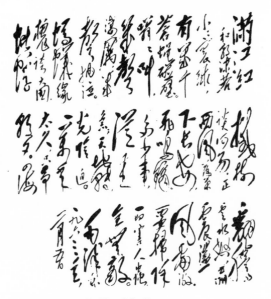

Reply to Comrade Kuo Mo-Jo

to the Melody of Man Chiang Hung

On this tiny globe
A few flies dash themselves against the wall,
Humming without cease,
Sometimes shrilling,
Sometimes moaning.
Ants on the locust tree assume a great nation swagger
And mayflies lightly plot to topple the giant tree.
The west wind scatters leaves over Changan,
And the arrows are flying, twanging.

So many deeds cry out to be done,
And always urgently;
The world rolls on,
Time presses.
Ten thousand years are too long,
Seize the day, seize the hour!
The Four Seas are rising, clouds and waters raging,
The Five Continents are rocking, wind and thunder roaring.
Away with all pests!
Our force is irresistible.

Mao Tse-tung
9 January 1963

Contents

Introduction
by Edgar Snow

Dr Joshua Horn's account of his fifteen years as a surgeon, teacher and field medical worker in China is a revelatory and moving book. A man obviously of noble service, his writing impresses us with his own humility and simplicity in contrast to his thoughtful admiration of the people of China transformed, as he sees them, by a great revolution in their environment and thought.

A poor boy himself, who with difficulty won a medical education in England, Dr Horn took honours as a student and on graduation became a lecturer at Cambridge. Tempted there by the promise of a professorship, he turned it down in order to practice medicine in some way he hoped would help poor men become free. He was a humanist with political convictions he sought to express in professional action. After World War II, when he was a surgeon with the British army, he became an outstanding traumatologist at the Birmingham Hospital. Then, in 1954, he volunteered for work in China and uprooted himself and his family, to live in an old world turned upside down.

Dr Horn offers explanations, mainly in the form of a life closely shared with ordinary people, of how Chinese doctors combined theory with practice; how acupuncture, herbalism and traditional medicine are made to play their role along with modern methods; how a mass of 'peasant doctors', under the direction of mobile medical teams, are trained to diagnose common diseases and on occasion even perform emergency operations in areas inaccessible to hospitals or clinics; how doctors benefit from some manual labour; how the system profits from group consultation, research and experience, in a changing land where highly trained doctors are still in short supply; and how the teachings of Mao Tse-tung are used to encourage and inspire whole communes and even the meekest citizen with hope and a will to act and to serve. By such means China's medical workers have, he asserts, conquered or brought under control epidemic diseases, syphilis, leprosy and schistosomiasis; advanced the treatment of severe burns and the reimplantation of severed limbs to the highest levels; won peasant support for planned parenthood; and become first in the world to create synthetic protein (insulin).

Dr Horn leaves no doubt that he himself is a believer in the effectiveness of Mao's Thought, but he makes no claims for miracles performed by it. His is no critical report, yet he frankly describes the difficult conditions of work and the material poverty which surrounded him. 'But in my experience', he writes, 'very few Chinese regard themselves as being poor. . . . The Chinese people have a richer cultural life, are more articulate, use their leisure time more profitably, and have a clearer understanding of where they want to go and how they are going to get there, than any people I have ever met. That makes them rich, not poor.' Evidently Dr Horn has made no gold for himself in China and yet clearly he also feels, as a result of his experience there, 'rich, not poor'.

1
Prelude

When I was a medical student in the early 1930s the curriculum was strictly divided into two parts. For three years we studied biochemistry, anatomy and physiology. Then for three years we walked the wards, learning the practice of clinical medicine. In retrospect, this separation of theory and practice was most unsatisfactory for the second half of the course seemed to have little connection with the first.

I enjoyed my preclinical studies and managed to collect various prizes and medals which helped keep the wolf from the door. I was short of money for my father was often unemployed, and in those days scholarships were few and niggardly in amount. I earned what I could by teaching and by doing manual work whenever I had the opportunity, but unemployment was widespread and it was not easy to find odd jobs.

I was disappointed that we had no contact with patients but I knew that this would come later on and that then we would be able to use the knowledge we had been accumulating.

I particularly enjoyed anatomy for the human body is constructed with exquisite ingenuity and dissection not only reveals the present stage reached in evolution, but also gives fascinating glimpses of the long process of adaptation and modification which has preceded it. Many structures which became useless as Man evolved, were not discarded but were adapted so that they could play an entirely new role.

The cadavers which we dissected mostly came from the workhouses and they bore all the signs of a life of hardship and deprivation.

Influenced by my father and by the militant struggles of the working class, I entered into the political life of the college, found myself moving towards the left and joined the Socialist Medical Association. Hitler, newly installed in power, was dragging Germany into the depths of savagery and J. B. S. Haldane, a geneticist of renown, with a towering intellect and unshakeable integrity, thundered warnings in the college quadrangle about the rise of Fascism in Germany and at home. Mosley's blackshirts, as arrogant and brutalized as their Nazi models, strutted through the streets of London and fanned flames of racial hatred. The number of unemployed rose steadily; poverty, hunger and insecurity affected the lives of millions.

A great deal of effort was expended in deciding what was the minimum level on which the underpaid workers could live. The British Medical Association appointed an expert committee to determine the nutritional state of the British people and although it set a standard slightly lower than that officially prescribed for Scottish convict prisons, it came to the conclusion that twenty per cent of the entire population lived at or below this level. The Ministry of Health rejected the findings of the British Medical Association on the remarkable grounds that the standard they had set was too high!

Indignant at the wrongness of it all, and wishing to understand and perhaps to influence events, some of us formed a college Socialist Society—now a commonplace but then, in my own college, an unheard-of act of rebellion. A young economics lecturer, Hugh Gaitskell, joined the Society. We had one meeting, harmless as it seemed to me, and then the Society was banned by the Provost. Most of us were flattered by being thought dangerous enough to ban and, with open contempt for authority, we continued to meet in the public house across the road. But Hugh Gaitskell left us, never to return.

Towards the end of 1932, the first of the Hunger Marchers converged on London to protest and win public support. They were contingents of angry, footsore, unemployed workers from all over the country and especially from the 'depressed areas' in Scotland, Wales and the North of England. I have a vivid recollection of a mass meeting of welcome in Hyde Park for it was the first time I experienced unprovoked police brutality. The Government had mobilized the Special Constables to take over regular police duties, so as to be able to concentrate large numbers of regular police in the Park. Without warning they charged into the peaceful demonstration, the mounted police trampling people underfoot, swinging their batons with the utmost viciousness.

The following Sunday, when sympathetic Londoners demonstrated in Trafalgar Square in support of the unemployed, the police made further charges, injuring and arresting hundreds.

We medicals in the college Socialist Society saw the Hunger March as an opportunity to give full play to our political convictions and medical knowledge. We set up first aid posts and organized teams to go to the collecting points and the dosshouses where the Hunger Marchers lodged, to treat their ailments and bolster up their morale. I doubt whether we did any good in either respect. Our professional skill was almost non-existent for so far we had dealt only with corpses and test-tubes. We swotted up something about the treatment of blisters, bunions and flat feet but, as it turned out, the men were more troubled by lice and haemorrhoids and they knew more about these than we did. As for bolstering up their morale, they had marched hundreds of miles and suffered great hardships while those who lacked determination had already dropped out. We, on the other hand, had suffered little more than the disapproval of our fellow students. Politically we thought that we ranged from the deepest red to the palest pink, but in truth, none of us had a clear idea what it was all about. We felt awkward in front of these unemployed miners, dockers and steel workers. We did not speak their language and they did not speak ours. Although we did not benefit them, I think they helped us. I still recall my sense of incongruity when I returned home after a session at the Shoreditch Baths and my mother gave me a succulent kipper for tea. A few hours before, we had handed out plates of bread and margarine to the marchers, feeling pious as we did so. The kipper lost its fragrance as I thought of the contrast and I realized that if my convictions were ever going to mean anything, they would have to be based on understanding rather than emotion, would have to go much deeper and express themselves more concretely than they did at that time, and I should have to find some way to break through the barriers which separated me from the industrial workers.

Shortly after passing my examinations in the basic medical sciences, and going over to the hospital for clinical training, I became dissatisfied with life as a medical student. This was partly because the lack of science in clinical work contrasted strikingly with the scientific nature of our studies in the first three years. I now see this was largely due to the attitude of our teachers, and to the organization of medical teaching. Our teachers, mostly well-fed, successful Harley Street specialists, went out of their way to deride our scientific aspirations and to extinguish any sparks of scientic inquiry which had been implanted in us. They had long since forgotten what they themselves had learned as junior medical students and they abjured us to do the same. Today matters are somewhat different, for medical schools are now largely staffed by full-time clinician/teachers whose work is divided between the training of medical students and clinical research. Partly as a result of this, science has penetrated much more deeply into clinical medicine than it had when I was a student. In those days our teachers were so-called 'honoraries', who gained large incomes from private practice and who used hospital appointments to consolidate their positions and increase their fame and fees. Students and hospital patients existed chiefly to secure these ends.

There were honourable exceptions to whom I shall always be grateful, but for the most part our clinical teachers were a miserable lot. They deeply resented any question, no matter how well-intentioned, if it did anything to reveal the sad, great gaps in their knowledge. I recall an occasion when I joined a teaching-ward round conducted by a physician who was famous both as a doyen of Harley Street, and as a pillar of the Church. He had an enormous income and he let it be known that he often talked directly with God (by appointment only). He took us to the bedside of a patient suffering from a disease which in those days was not only fatal, but was hardly possible to palliate. Without any regard for the patient's feelings, he gave us a long and pompous discourse on the condition and then, without the slightest hint that he could really do nothing of value, he told us exactly how to treat it. Treatment was begun on a Monday with one drop of arsenic solution. On Tuesday one gave two drops and so on, increasing by one drop a day until Sunday when, of course, one rested and gave no medicine. The next week saw the same process in reverse, reducing the amount of medicine by one drop daily. After three such cycles, all medicine was withheld for three weeks and then the process started again and continued until the inevitable end. I was so amazed at the extraordinary precision of this regime that I asked what evidence it was based on. A painful silence followed broken only by the suppressed giggling of a probationer nurse. The holy man, visibly nettled, looked upwards for guidance. He must have found it, for in tones of the deepest contempt, he said: 'Professor' (this was the nearest approach to name-calling that he ever permitted himself), 'I think you would perhaps find more profitable employment elsewhere', and he jerked his head towards the door.

This, perhaps, is a rather extreme example of the intellectual dishonesty and lack of modesty of our clinical teachers but most of them were characterized by a crude rule-of-thumb approach, by contempt for science and by a steadfast refusal to admit that there was a great deal about which they knew nothing. Another reason for my dissatisfaction was a feeling that I

13

was wasting the best years of my life and I rebelled against the prospect of continuing to do so for another three years. Full of youthful energy, I resented having to cram my head with empirical knowledge and dogma, pass one examination after another and scrape a living by whatever means were open to me. I resented my isolation from the mainstream of life, resented the fact that the ideas which effervesced in my mind had all to be put into cold storage until I secured my magic diploma, resented the fact that I was pawning my present for my future.

As I write this, here in Peking, China's Great Cultural Revolution is under way and hundreds of thousands of students are demanding that courses should be shortened, that examinations cease to be tests of memory and become tests of reasoning power and an aid to study, that methods of study should be revolutionized so as to link theory with practice, and that the isolation of students from the life of the people be ended by regular participation in ordinary work. They say that as things are, they waste the best years of their life. I can fully sympathize with their attitude for that is more or less how I felt thirty years earlier. The difference is that the students of China, firmly linked with the mass of the people, have it in their power to change things and are taking purposeful steps to do so, whereas I could make only some futile flurries.

At that time I liked reading Somerset Maugham. The fact that he had begun life as a medical student seemed to give us a common point of departure. One day it struck me that Somerset Maugham might hold the key to my own emancipation. I was not yet twenty and he, I thought, must by now be in an advanced stage of decrepitude. Surely he must find it difficult to travel to those distant, romantic islands? Surely he must be running short of material for future novels? I would propose a division of labour; I would do the travelling, and he the writing. I would interview the beachcombers, the drunkards, the enchantresses and the fallen missionaries; he would weave my bare reportage into tales of charm. He would secure the fame and fortune and I my freedom and my expenses.

I wrote him a letter explaining the proposition.

Maugham must have received hundreds of similar nonsensical yet burningly sincere letters, and it is to his credit that he answered. His reply was brief and to the point. He was not yet infirm and did not need a traveller by proxy, I should complete my medical studies and then, if I still wanted to travel, I might get a post as ship's surgeon. I was disgusted and threw away his letter. Nevertheless, I followed his advice. Had I not done so, perhaps I should never have travelled to China and would not now be writing this book.

After I had qualified I was invited to go to Cambridge to lecture in Anatomy. The newly appointed Professor of Anatomy, who had been my teacher, regarded himself as a kind of radical. He was determined to sweep away the cobwebs which had settled on the anatomy department in the University of Cambridge, and he knew he would encounter stiff opposition and would need allies in the struggles to come. I welcomed the prospect of a tussle with established authority and at the beginning of the Spring term, when the crocuses and daffodils were speckling the manicured college lawns, I took up residence in Cambridge and began to live the life of Reilly. Everything was

14

perfect. Cambridge was entrancingly beautiful in a heady, soigné way. The work was interesting and I found that I was able to evoke a response from my students. I attached myself to an experimental anatomist, assisted him in research work and learned much from him. My salary seemed to me to be munificent beyond the dreams of avarice for I could send half of it to my parents and live comfortably on the remainder. I rented a furnished flat over a garage and became, as I thought, a completely free and independent human being. A small garden at the back of the garage sloped down to a sidewater of the Cam, and a punt, moored here, went with the flat. Before going to bed, I would punt up the river past Queens' College, under Newton's bridge, alongside lawns that are to be found only in England, through the narrows beyond the Bridge of Sighs until, when it reaches Magdalene College, the Cam leaves fairyland and becomes an ordinary thoroughfare. Then I would drift back, envious of the courting couples on the lawns and enchanted by the fragrance of the jasmine and honeysuckle.

Once a week I was expected to dine in one of the College Halls; I then sat at the high table, and was waited on by a liveried butler. The food was heavy and plentiful while the old silver cutlery seemed even heavier and more plentiful. After dinner, fuzzy with doctored audit ale and rich old port, we would retire to the oak-panelled common room, to sip brandy and listen to the allegedly sparkling conversation of the Master and his cronies. At first I was duly impressed by the pomp and tradition, by the Georgian candle-sticks and by the gilt-framed oil paintings, so darkened by smoke from countless cigars and from the open log fire that one could scarcely make out their imperfections. Soon, however, it all began to pall. By mid-term the Master had used up his repertoire of witticisms and was now regaling us with stories we all knew by heart, but that nevertheless still evoked simulated laughter. It was unthinkable to leave the room before the Master had gone, yet I felt that if I remained I should surely say something indiscreet. The atmosphere was as cloying and sickly as the over-sweet port that is so highly esteemed in these circles. My mind would return to the Hunger Marchers in Shoreditch Baths, and I began to feel an impostor.

When the academic year ended, the Professor wanted me to stay and take up Anatomy as a career and tempted me with prospects of a chair within seven or eight years.

I was happy in Cambridge, and I wrestled long before deciding. But I had studied medicine in order to practise medicine, not to get a safe, cloistered post. There was an atmosphere of tenseness, of struggle, both in England and throughout the world. I felt that I was committed to the struggle and that it would be cowardly to wriggle out of it before I had engaged in it. I knew that after a few comfortable years in the enervating academic atmosphere of Cambridge, I would sink into a rut and find it difficult to leave.

I decided to seek house appointments in my own hospital in London, to specialize in surgery, and to work for the Fellowship of the Royal College of Surgeons.

But first, before settling down to a long, hard grind, remembering Somerset Maugham's advice, I signed on as a ship's surgeon in a cargo boat bound for China and the Far East.

2

A glimpse of China

We sailed from the Pool of London at dawn on Christmas Day, 1936. My British shipmates were disgruntled at having to leave on Christmas Day and many of them had hangovers from consolatory junketings in the Galleons Inn the night before. But the Chinese crew were glad to be leaving this land of cold and fog and to be sailing back to their homes and families.

I stood on deck, so excited at the prospect of a great adventure that I paid no heed to the biting wind as fussy tugs nosed us out into the tideway and as we slipped down London's great river, past forests of cranes, past warehouses crammed with strange goods exuding smells which I could not recognize, past breweries giving off a fragrance which I could recognize all too easily, past ships from all over the world, past the pompous magnificence of Greenwich until, imperceptibly, the river became an estuary and the estuary became the sea.

Then the movement of the ship felt different. We no longer glided; we thrust our way forward and the wind and the waves tried to hold us back. The powerful old engines throbbed and sent a tremor through the ship as we gained speed and carved our way through the grey sea.

Under the captain, the undisputed master of the ship, were three main departments, deck, engine room and stewarding, with two minor departments, radio and medical. Between the three main departments there was intense rivalry and mutual dislike.

With the exception of the third officer, I got on very well with my shipmates. He, however, became my mortal enemy. He was a racist, a fascist, a braggart and a snob. He had acquired some kind of public-school accent and he threw his weight about insufferably. The Spanish Civil War was on and as we sailed down the coast of Spain towards Gibraltar we spotted some British destroyers engaged in enforcing the farce of 'non-intervention', which meant prohibiting aid from reaching the legal Spanish Republican Government while Hitler and Mussolini poured in a stream of weapons for their protégé, General Franco. The Third Officer gloated: 'Franco will teach those bastards a lesson. He may use coloured troops but he knows how to handle them and he himself is a Christian and a Gentleman. Hitler will never let him down. We could do with a Hitler in England to keep the wogs and the upstarts in their place!'

At first I tried reasoning with him but we had no common ground and we drifted into enmity. Needless to say his hatred for coloured people didn't stop him from whoring with native girls in every port of call. But, on one occasion, it proved to be a stronger force than his phoney patriotism. The Italian invasion of Ethiopia was recent history and feeling still ran very high against the barbarities committed in the name of Mussolini's 'civilizing mission'. When we arrived in Shanghai, we found an Italian and a British warship there and one evening their crews engaged in a regular battle—ostensibly around the issue of the invasion of Ethiopia. Normally, the Third Officer would have been delighted to see the Italians get badly beaten up but on this occasion he supported them and said that 'we' had a lot to learn from Mussolini.

A few years later the ship was torpedoed and sunk by one of Hitler's submarines. I do not know if any of my shipmates perished but, by an extraordinary quirk of fate, I know that the Third Officer did not. Nearly twenty-eight years after my voyage as ship's surgeon, while on holiday in a North China seaside resort, I visited a nearby port where my ship had called. Walking along the jetty in the bright morning sunshine, my companions and I saw a British ship tied up alongside. One of the ship's officers must have heard us talking English for he came down the gangplank to engage us in conversation. He was big, burly, red-faced, wore his cap at a rakish angle, spoke with a public-school accent and although it was not yet ten in the morning, he was swaying on his heels exhaling a fruity aroma of gin. It was my old enemy the Third Officer.

He had not the slightest idea who I was and at first I wasn't quite sure about him. He asked us aboard to have a little drink, but I thought that time could have done nothing to bring us closer and I declined.

The daily ship's inspection took us into the Chinese crew's quarters and I was shocked at the contrast between their living conditions and ours. Whereas the officers each had a cabin on deck, the Chinese crew were huddled together in the after part of the ship just above the propeller. Their quarters were hot, noisy and cramped but they kept them very clean.

Although their accommodation was poor, their food was much more appetizing than our own and I sometimes conducted a one-man 'hygiene inspection' of the Chinese galley at meal times. When the Chinese cook sensed that my interests extended beyond the purely medical, he usually offered me a bowl of some tasty concoction and showed me how to use chopsticks. Then I would sit round on the after deck with the Chinese sailors, show my approval of their cooking by sign language and try to make contact with them. A few of them could speak English and from them I gradually acquired some understanding of the intense exploitation from which they suffered. They nearly all came from the big Southern ports where overcrowding and poverty were acute. Jobs on foreign-going ships were highly sought after for the wages were comparatively good and, at least for the duration of the voyage, they were secure. Consequently an opportunity existed for their exploiter's hangers-on to squeeze something for themselves and this was utilized to the full. In order to be considered for a job at sea, applicants had to bribe layers of brokers, middlemen, compradors and agents of all nationalities. To do this, they either had to borrow the bribe money or sign an undertaking to pay it off out of their wages at compound interest. In this way they lost the greater part of their wages before they saw a penny of it and since they usually signed over most of the remainder to their families, they themselves actually received very little in cash. Ah Li, my medical assistant, who kept the sick bay spick-and-span and dusted the regulation twelve Winchester quarts of medicine, found himself in possession of ten shillings as we neared the home port and he planned to use it to buy his little boy a tricycle. I doubted whether he could buy a tricycle for so little money but he assured me that it was sufficient and so it turned out to be, for in one

17

of our ports of call, he bought a sturdy little Japanese-made tricycle which we parked in my cabin. As the ship slowly came alongside in Shanghai, Ah Li spotted his wife on the quayside holding their baby son in her arms. He rushed into my cabin, more excited than I had ever seen him, seized the tricycle and held it aloft for his son to see. When the child realized the treasure in store for him, he almost flew through the air to get it and the parents' delight at the child's happiness made it a most moving reunion.

In Shanghai, the old crew was paid off and a new crew signed on. When the applicants had bribed, cajoled and squeezed their way through all obstacles, they still had to cross the medical hurdle. A rigorous medical selection had already taken place before I saw them, for most of the men had sailed before and none of them was prepared to squander bribe money if there was no chance of passing the medical test. Nevertheless I could feel the tension as the men lined up for examination; their future, the future of their families, whether they would eat or go hungry, whether they would sleep with a roof over their heads or doss down on the waterfront, depended on the result of my examination. I had always known that medicine cannot be divorced from social conditions but now, at the very beginning of my medical career, I was confronted by the contradiction between health, exploitation and poverty in a particularly naked form. In the crowded conditions aboard ship it would be easy for a man with open TB to infect a dozen others during a voyage and I therefore regarded the detection of infectious diseases as my main duty. I took this, my first real medical undertaking, very seriously and tackled it slowly and thoroughly. This irritated some of the officers who wanted to get ashore to the delights of Shanghai and they urged me to get a move on, telling me of previous ship's surgeons who had done the whole job in a couple of hours. But I plodded on, conscious of my lack of experience and of the serious consequences of making a mistake. Many of the men had evidence of vitamin deficiency diseases but unless their symptoms were severe, I usually passed them, for with good food they would recover within a few weeks and they presented no danger to their shipmates. I rejected men with active venereal disease, but I passed those with small ruptures for this was their only chance to save enough money to get them operated on, while if, by chance, they strangulated at sea, I would be able to deal with them surgically.

In spite of my somewhat lenient requirements, I examined more than two hundred applicants in order to select eighty. This will give some idea of the poor state of health even among skilled sea-faring men.

Although it is more than thirty years since I first went ashore in Shanghai, some scenes, some impressions of the week I spent there are indelibly etched on my mind.

The beggars. The swarms of beggars of all ages, whole and diseased, vociferous and silent, hopeful and hopeless, blind and seeing. All having in common their poverty, their degradation.

The prostitutes. The smart ones in the foreign concessions with make-up, high-heeled shoes and skin-tight dresses slit to the thigh. The cheap ones in the sailors' districts, unkempt, raucous, brazen, The child prostitutes. The two frightened, bewildered little girls dragged along, one in each hand, by their owner who offered them singly or together for fifty cents an hour.

The poverty. The rows of matsheds where hundreds of thousands lived and died. The hunger-swollen bellies. The rummaging in garbage bins for possible scraps of food.

The children. I can do no better than quote a Canadian hotelier who lived in pre-Liberation Shanghai for more than twenty years and who, on a return visit in 1965, recalled the familiar sights of old Shanghai:[1]

'I searched for scurvy-headed children. Lice-ridden children. Children with inflamed red eyes. Children with bleeding gums. Children with distended stomachs and spindly arms and legs. I searched the sidewalks day and night for children who had been purposely deformed by beggars. Beggars who would leech on to any well-dressed passer-by to blackmail sympathy and offerings, by pretending the hideous-looking child was their own.

'I looked for children covered with horrible sores upon which flies feasted. I looked for children having a bowel movement, which, after much strain, would only eject tapeworms.

'I looked for child slaves in alleyway factories. Children who worked twelve hours a day, literally chained to small press punches. Children who, if they lost a finger, or worse, often were cast into the streets to beg and forage in garbage bins for future subsistence.'

In 1965 he searched without finding, but in the 1930s there was no need to search far for such sights for everywhere to be seen.

Rewi Alley, New Zealand writer and poet, for many years chief inspector of factories in Shanghai, wrote:

'I think back on the eleven years of factory inspection in Shanghai, and of all the crude exploitation seen. The long lines of weeping children, many only nine or ten, stirring the basins of silk cocoons in silk filatures, the dead-weary apprentices with beri-beri swollen legs in the dark sweat shops of back alley-ways, the exploited contract labour working their twelve-hour shifts in cotton mills, and all the rest of the filthy oppression the system brought in its train. Then the end of the road for prostitutes thrown up by an utterly wicked society, whose life amongst the cheap brothels on Foochow Road averaged two years. The callous, bloated rich and the incredible poverty of the poor.'

The bodies floating down the river. Leaning against the ship rail, I could see them bobbing up and down in the murky water, now hitching against a buoy or a mooring rope; now breaking free to continue their journey down to the Peaceful Ocean. I asked the bosun whose bodies they were, where they had come from. He shrugged. Not with indifference but with resignation and with great sadness. 'Who knows? All are different. Some just died but no money for burial. Some jumped into the river out of great sorrow. Some were thrown in by their enemies. There is famine up the river and many thousands die each day. There are bandits. There are soldiers who are no different from bandits. These days, many girls are sold into the Houses of Joy and some prefer the river. China is sick and that is why there are many bodies in the river.'

The wealth. Ostentatious, overflowing wealth. Shop fronts of onyx and stainless steel. Shop windows crammed with diamonds and gold. The Longest

[1] W. H. Scott, *Eastern Horizon, Vol. V. No. 6. June 1966*

Bar in the world where a Tom Collins cost more than a labourer could earn in a month; where women flashed rings that would ransom thousands from death and desolation.

The rickshaw races. Fat foreigners from many countries, straw-hatted and sweating, choosing their pullers. Poking them in the ribs to size them up. Lining them up for the start. All fair and square. Nothing crooked about this type of race, good fun. Once the length of the Bund. Barely a mile. A dollar for the winner and fifty cents for the runner-up. Pretty generous when you come to think of it. The pullers. Straining every muscle, gasping for breath, half-naked bodies dripping with sweat.

The Great World. The biggest, noisiest, most extraordinary amusement centre in existence. Snacks and drinks to tickle every palate. Shops selling everything imaginable and unimaginable. Peking opera competing with leg shows, acrobatics with strip-tease, magicians with mademoiselles. All jostling one another, all screaming for customers, all itching to empty your pockets. I did not know it then, but I was in the heart of the empire of Tu Yueh-sheng, leader of the Green Gang secret society of which Chiang Kai-shek was a member, unofficial Mayor of Shanghai, King of Shanghai's pimps, drug peddlers and brothel keepers, holder of more directorates of Chinese banks and business houses than any other man in Shanghai, decorated by Chiang Kai-shek, owner of a private army of fifteen thousand armed thugs, a multi-millionaire gangster listed in China's 'Who's Who' for 1930 as banker, philanthropist and welfare worker.

Imperialism. Shanghai, the greatest city of a sovereign country, with warships from every country moored in her main artery, their sailors roaming the streets at will, a law unto themselves. The city was sliced up into the International and French concessions, both enjoying extraterritoriality. Criminals had only to cross the concession boundary to escape the law, but an unwritten agreement stipulated that suspected communists would be handed over on request. The police officers were foreigners and the ordinary Chinese policemen under their command wore foreign-type uniforms. I went to the British Bank on the waterfront to cash a cheque for £10. A huge, imposing building with granite pillars and flights of marble steps. At the top, bearded Sikhs holding rifles with fixed bayonets guarded great bronze doors. I felt that I must have made a mistake, they could not possibly cash cheques for £10 here. So I asked the Sikh guard, and while I did so, a Chinese peddler sneaked past, hoping to sell his cigarettes inside. The Sikh spotted him, thrust a rifle butt viciously into his loins, and kicked him down the marble stairs. 'Sorry, sir,' he explained, 'they think they own the place!'

The Chinese certainly owned Shanghai, but they were not to take possession for another twelve years.

Within a few days of leaving Shanghai to continue our voyage northward, one of the crew reported sick with fever, pains in the limbs and severe headache. I could find no cause for his illness, so I put him to bed. I instructed Ah Li to feed and nurse him, and I visited him twice a day. The sick bay was stocked, according to Board of Trade regulations, with twelve Winchester quarts of medicines. They were labelled, I supposed, according to the diseases they were alleged to cure. One bottle, however, was described as 'Sweating

Mixture', and I was not sure whether it was to cure or to cause sweating. I tried a dose and concluded it was either aspirin or something similar. Then I gave some to the patient, and although it eased his headache, the fever continued and his general condition gradually deteriorated. He became weak, refused all food and his mind became clouded. On the third day I noticed a faint rash on his chest, and a slight distension of the abdomen. I suspected typhoid fever, and decided to keep him isolated until we reached the next port. As we sailed into harbour I took a blood sample, and sent it ashore for urgent examination. Within a few hours the report came; he was suffering not from typhoid fever, but from typhus fever. In this part of the world the two diseases resemble one another so closely that, if one asks for a blood test for one of them, the laboratory also carries out a test for the other.

The patient was put ashore and taken to the hospital for infectious diseases, where, as I was later informed, he made a good recovery. But he created all sorts of complications for the ship. Typhus fever is carried by lice, and if there were infected lice on board, not only could there be a danger of the disease spreading among the crew but, much more serious for the quarantine authorities, we were a source of danger to every port where we docked. Unless and until I could issue a certificate declaring that this danger did not exist, we would not be allowed to go alongside and no one would be allowed ashore.

The lice were the key to the situation. If there were no lice, there was no danger.

I assembled the crew on deck and, assisted by Ah Li, systematically examined their quarters, bedding and clothing. We did not find a single louse. Then I asked the crew to strip, and I examined their bodies with similar negative results. We then inspected the officers and their quarters in the same way, finally Ah Li and I examined one another. Only the Fascist-minded Third Officer refused to be inspected, saying that since he never went near the 'yellow bastards', he 'could not have got their bloody lice'. But, when I pointed out that we had not found any lice on the Chinese, and, maybe, he had given them his 'bloody lice', he reluctantly agreed.

Since there were no lice on the ship, the sick sailor must have been infected before joining and must have been incubating the disease when I examined him. I signed a statement to this effect, and the Port Sanitary Officer, after a perfunctory search, countersigned it. We were then allowed to go alongside and tie-up after large metal rat discs, which would preclude a rat from running along the ropes to the quay, had been fixed to the mooring lines.

The next port was a dismal looking place, which served as an outlet for a British-owned coal-mine. We took on enough coal here to last us for the rest of the voyage and during the loading I obtained an idea of current rates of pay for Chinese labourers.

I watched the tall, lean North Chinese carrying coal several hundred yards from the dump. Working in pairs, they would fill a heavy wicker basket, take it up the ship's side, tip the coal into the bunkers, and be paid for the trip as they left the gangplank. The rate was one cash a trip between the two men. This worked out at one-fiftieth of a penny a trip a man, at the current rate of exchange. Since one round trip took about ten minutes, a man was unlikely to get in more than fifty trips a day, for which he would get the equivalent of one penny. It is possible this could buy enough coarse grain to keep a man alive, but what their families lived on, or what happened when there was no ship in port, can only be imagined.

As we sailed North, the weather became colder and the sea lost its blueness. We had travelled through tropical seas for several weeks and, while I had an adequate supply of white cotton uniforms, I lacked cold weather clothing. Soon it became exceptionally cold. It was February, and by the time we reached Dairen, ice was floating on the sea. The steam pipes had not been lagged, and as soon as we docked, they froze and we were left without heating in our cabins, without hot water and tasted scarcely any hot food. Gloom descended.

We were loading soya bean oil in bulk, a difficult task that necessitated the re-arrangement of all the other cargo. This was the Chief Officer's responsibility and he groaned under the weight of it. He insisted on doing everything himself and complained that no one helped him. His lady friend, a White Russian emigrée of whom he had been speaking throughout the voyage, did not appear as expected, and he had no time to go ashore. The weather got colder and colder and gradually he worked himself into a state of acute anxiety. One afternoon, when his steward went to his cabin with a cup of tea, he found the door locked on the inside, the port holes tightly screwed down and no answer to his vigorous banging. There was nothing for it but to smash the door, and this was done in the nick of time. The distraught Chief Officer, determined to get warm and forget his troubles, had brought two charcoal burners into his cabin and had gone to bed with the cat. The animal was already dead from carbon monoxide fumes given off by the smouldering charcoal and the Chief Officer was unconscious and breathing irregularly. I carried him out on deck, gave him artificial respiration, and warmed him with hot water bottles while Ah Li rushed ashore to get an ambulance. Within half an hour we were racing through the streets of Dairen to the City Hospital.

Dairen was then a Japanese colony, and the hospital was staffed by Japanese doctors and nurses. I remember that it was intensely hot, with an overpowering stench of garlic. Going into the hospital from the bitterly cold, windswept streets, was like entering an oven, with the heat accentuated by the crowds of people inside, all chewing garlic, which was thought to protect against respiratory tract infections.

The Chief Officer developed pneumonia, but he recovered with sulpha drugs and with a form of wave therapy greatly favoured by the Japanese doctors. We had to sail without him, but he caught an aeroplane to Singapore in time to rejoin the ship on the homeward journey.

The Japanese colonialists were arrogant and overbearing towards their imperialist rivals, but they treated the Chinese with viciousness. Curses, kicks and lashes were distributed liberally on the slightest provocation, or even on none at all, and it was easy to sense the smouldering hatred the brutality aroused. At that time, in that place, the Chinese were powerless to resist, but elsewhere in China the Communist armies were regrouping after their heroic Long March, and a weapon was being forged which, in eight years, would smash the mighty Japanese military machine and humble the arrogant conquerors.

On our return journey we again called at Shanghai, and a passenger, who had left the ship there a few weeks earlier, sent me an invitation to a banquet.

It was my first experience of the delights of first-class Chinese cooking, and even after all these years I recall the procession of crisp sucking pig, mandarin fish, plovers' eggs, roast duck, truffles and soups of surpassing delicacy. Whenever it seemed that the end had been reached, and gluttony had been subdued, a momentary pause in the succession of dishes signalled the appearance of a culinary tour-de-force which began the whole process over again.

Late at night the party came to an end and I began my walk towards the ship. The streets were quiet, deserted, and a gusty sea wind drove rain clouds across the moon. From round a corner came the sound of marching feet. Soldiers appeared, escorting a young man, stripped to the waist, his hands tied behind him, his hair tousled and his face bruised and swollen. He marched with pride as though leading the soldiers.

When I reached the boatman who would row me out to the ship, I asked him what was the meaning of the strange procession. The young man, he said, was a Communist or at least, he might be one. In any event, he would be shot since he was under suspicion. There were such processions every night; sometimes many.

As the boatman rowed me across the swift, dark waters of the Whangpoo, I could see his family huddling in the bottom of the boat which was their home and their source of livelihood. A few flimsy planks separated them from the turbulent river, a few coins saved them from starvation. I thought of the unseen bodies floating down the river. I thought of the pain, the misery, and the degradation that was China. I thought of the contrast between the meal I had just eaten and the gnawing hunger of millions of Chinese. 'They must rise up,' I said to myself. 'They must rise in revolution. A vast, searing revolution that will destroy all the evil, the oppression, the brutality, so that they can build anew!'

What I did not know was that in the vast hinterland, in the hovels of the treaty ports, in the sweatshops and foreign-owned mines, on remote mountain sides, the revolution was already seething and gaining strength; that the Chinese people had already found leaders on whom they could rely; that the young man holding high his bruised, battered head as he marched to the execution ground was typical of countless thousands of anonymous heroes who in the end were to win victory for the revolution.

3

'Quick! Thy tablets, Memory'

It was to be seventeen years before I returned to China. Seventeen years in which the whole world changed and in which China changed most of all.

The Second World War had come and gone and nothing ever could be the same again.

During the blitz I had worked as a surgeon in the dockside area of London, spending night after night operating on air-raid casualties while bombs rained down and buildings blazed. In the mornings, before snatching a few hours' sleep, I would glance outside at the results of the holocaust and would always be astonished to find that much remained standing between the smouldering ruins, and to see the indomitable dockers in their cloth caps going off to work as if nothing had happened.

Then four years in the Army, now compressed into a hotchpotch of vague recollections with a few vivid impressions standing out like poppies in a field of corn.

The Second Front—the Allied landings on the coast of Normandy at last materializing after months of waiting, drilling and marching in lush country-side which, though unkempt, flowered and flourished despite the absence of civilians. Surely the English spring has never been more beautiful than in that memorable year of 1944!

A padre in my unit, unnerved by the waiting, the uncertainty, the contrast between present beauty and the prospect of unknown danger, put a bullet through his head. We went on arguing, playing poker, listening to the radio and marching. Then, long after we could pitch our tents and unpack our equipment blindfold, we went over.

Grape-fruit juice and real butter on the American tank-landing craft that took us across! Forgotten delights!

Through the surf into the fields of Normandy.

As I write, a torrent of memories comes flooding back, clamouring for space on pages not meant for them. Mostly they are of food or war.

Little copses of wooden crosses sprouting up wherever we pitched our tents and worked for a few days. I had seen many of those who lay beneath the crosses die.

The anaesthetist killed by my side while I was operating. So quickly, so quietly. A mortar bomb fragment tore a tiny hole in the canvas over us, went into his brain and he was dead. An orderly picked up the bottle of ether and kept the patient asleep while I finished the operation.

The galaxy of mushrooms growing in the rich, untended Norman fields, as close-packed as the stars in the Milky Way. With my tent-mate, a first-class cook, I would go out at dawn and fill an Army pack with button mushrooms, disdaining those past their prime. Then at night, over a primus stove, he would fry a duck, 'liberated' from a deserted farm-house and cook the mushrooms in duck-fat. Our ridge tent would be full of smoke, for black-out regulations forbade us to lift the flap. He taught me to make potato crisps that don't stick together. Then, with friends armed with bottles of excavated Calvados, we shared midnight feasts.

When it was peaceful, it seemed as though the peace were absolute and eternal. But when the war roared and raged, it rent the heavens, stripped the leaves from the trees and it seemed as though peace could never return.

My operating shift started at 4 a.m. and I had to struggle to swallow slivers of luke-warm, naked-pink soya sausage.

Later, when our supplies ran out, I was sent into the Falaise gap, where French resistance fighters were locked in bitter combat with encircled German troops, to establish a medical aid post for the French. That night, after setting up the post, I went in search of the local Resistance leaders. I found the building to which I had been directed. All was dark. The windows and doors on the ground floor had been blown in. I entered, flicked my torch into empty, ruined rooms and started to go upstairs. A gun was pressed into my back. The Resistance were on the look-out for a collaborator who had betrayed many of them to the Gestapo and they were taking no chances. When I had established my identity, I was taken to an upper room where resistance fighters were sleeping, close-packed on the floor. After a brief discussion on the military situation and its medical needs, we started talking politics. They produced a few pamphlets by Lenin and Stalin, so worn and dog-eared that they were scarcely legible. They were youths who had grown to manhood under the Nazi occupation and they were groping their way towards a deeper understanding of the ugly world into which they had been born. We talked all through the night. They were the survivors of a much larger number who had fallen before Nazi firing-squads or had been tortured to death. They yearned for a better world after their national foe had been defeated and they were looking for the way to build it.

I, too, was feeling my way forward politically.

In Holland we took over a German hospital for high-ranking Nazi naval officers. The low quality of surgical treatment in use shocked me and I wondered how the ordinary German soldiers fared. Yet only a quarter of a century earlier, before the Nazis had mutilated German science and destroyed her best scientists, Germany had led the world in surgery. I was angered by the swaggering arrogance of the captured Nazi officers. They strutted about in their gold braid, Iron Crosses and jack-boots and had the impudence to demand that only pure Aryan blood be transfused into their wounded compatriots. They were, however, easily deflated by a few sharply issued commands.

The war finished and I resumed my career as a civilian surgeon—not in London where I had always lived until I joined the Army, but in Birmingham. My experience in the treatment of air-raid casualties and as a military surgeon had given me a great interest in the treatment of injuries and Birmingham had the only hospital in the country devoted exclusively to the treatment of injuries. I worked there for seven years. My family started to grow up. I had a contract for life as a consultant surgeon in the National Health Service. I seemed destined to spend the rest of my days as a surgical specialist in Britain's second city.

Then, in 1954, we uprooted ourselves and went to China en famille. Apart from a few home visits we have lived in China ever since.

I will not go into the numerous reasons behind our decision to go to China. Foremost among them was the political reason. I had glimpsed the old China, I knew that in 1949 the Communist armies had finally liberated the whole of the mainland and that now the Chinese people were engaged in the enormous task of building a modern Socialist state on the ruins of one that had been half feudal and half colonial. I was on China's side. I ardently wished to contribute what little skill I had to an heroic undertaking which would change the face of China and of the world.

One event which crystallized our decision was when my wife and I saw a film of the construction of a dam across the Huai river, part of a gigantic scheme of flood control. Hundreds of thousands of peasants scurried about carrying baskets of earth or stones on bamboo carrying-poles. A shot showed a group of peasants tamping the earth with a huge stone. Time after time the stone thudded down. A close-up showed it striking the earth and also showed the peasants' feet. Their feet were bare.

My wife and I looked at each other. She voiced my thought when she said, 'They need plenty of accident surgeons there.'

I do not wish to give the impression that our coming to China was in any way based on humanitarianism. Most of the world's peasants work in bare feet and yet we never thought of going to any country except China. It was a question of how, in a particular situation, one could make one's best political contribution.

Ever since my student days my political convictions had been getting stronger and more firmly based in Marxist theory. I had never wished to be an armchair theoretician, but a combination of circumstances sharply restricted my opportunities for political work. I knew that China was at the crest of an upsurge of the people and that events there would have a direct impact on every other country in the world, including my own.

Our 'plane touched down in Peking—not at the new enmarbled International airport but at the homely little airport, no longer used, near the Summer Palace. We had to wait a few hours for some other arrivals, and from the moment of landing we felt enveloped equally by the warmth of the autumn sunshine and by the friendship of the people. No stiletto-heeled, charm-trained air hostesses here! Just pig-tailed girls with rosy cheeks who smiled because they were happy and who made guests feel welcome because they liked them. One of them caught a praying-mantis for my six year old daughter, and tied a length of plastic thread from one of her braids round the insect's leg so that the little girl could play with it and feel at home.

We have been in China for fifteen years. Fifteen years of immersion in the tasks of the present; of study; of progressive identification with the road taken by the Chinese people; of deepening appreciation of their great qualities and of their outstanding leaders; of change in our environment and in ourselves, sometimes imperceptible, sometimes sharp and painful; of slowly growing understanding of the laws governing the movement of society. Now I rummage into the recesses of my memory and recapture some of my early impressions.

26

Inevitably they are tinged with a hindsight which I shall allow to emerge whenever it makes things clearer, for I am only gradually coming to realize that beneath China's calm exterior, there have been tensions, currents and cross currents, an unseen implacable struggle. These are being revealed by the Cultural Revolution which, as I write, colours and dominates all one's thoughts and actions.

A few days after arriving in China I watched the National Day Parade on October 1st. I had never before experienced such a mass demonstration of unity, joy and confidence. Half a million marched and one and a half million watched. Chairman Mao and other Party and government leaders, distinguished guests from abroad and what are called in China, 'democratic personages' which means Chinese who are not in the Party but who are representatives of progressive strata of the Chinese people, stood on the marble balustrade atop the massive, red-ochre Gate of Heavenly Peace and reviewed the parade.

Block after block of workers, peasants, students, professional workers of all kinds and ordinary Peking residents marched proudly by, carrying banners, scarlet flags, models of everything from locomotives to outsize turnips, statistics of what they had accomplished and what they intended to accomplish. Some of the peasants were a little undisciplined. They had come a long way to see their beloved Chairman and they wanted more than a fleeting glimpse of him. So when they saw him, they stopped, waved and shouted and the Chairman waved back.

The military contingents, impressively precise in their marching, carried weapons of an excellence that contrasted strikingly with their simple cotton uniforms, devoid of badges of rank, epaulettes or decorations. . . . A few years later, this suddenly changed. The armymen appeared in smart gaberdine with shining leather belts and straps, badges of rank, epaulettes, medals, peaked caps and all the trappings of the type of Army with which we are familiar in the West. No one knew why. Some said it was a sign of increasing prosperity. Others that it was inevitable that the People's Liberation Army should sooner or later come into line with other armies, including the Soviet army. Some of us were not too happy about it. The army that had marched eight thousand miles from the South-East to the North-West of China, that had torn the guts out of the mighty Japanese Imperial Army, that, armed with millet and rifles and an invincible, militant, revolutionary ideology, had defeated a Kuomintang army of eight million bristling with the best that the US could produce, had worn simple cotton uniforms, cloth shoes, and no distinctions of rank. Why start these things now? At the time we did not know the answer but now we know that it reflected the struggle between the capitalist and socialist line in military affairs. The capitalist line, in a nutshell, was to rely chiefly on weapons, equipment, military discipline and training; the socialist line was to give first place to the unity between the army and people, the unity between soldiers and commanders and, above all, to the political consciousness and self-imposed discipline of every soldier, sailor and airman.

After prolonged struggles, the socialist line of Chairman Mao won out and the Chinese army today again wears cotton uniforms, has no distinction of officer rank and is the most politically conscious army in the world.

One of the remaining impressions from my first National Day parade is of the music. Knowing only a vulgarized Western version, I had expected that Chinese music would be incomprehensible or even repulsive to me. It was not so. When I first heard the swelling chords of the 'East turns Red' fill the huge square, the sweetness and majesty of the melody evoked a very strong response. But the tune that really gripped me by the throat was the old army song which bears the cumbersome title 'Three Principles of Discipline and Eight Points for Attention'. It is a jolly jingle of great verve and zest which draws its power from its associations. It is as much a part of the People's Liberation Army as the simple red star on the soldiers' floppy cloth caps. It originated way back in the 1930s when most armymen were illiterate peasants. Until then, practically every army that the Chinese people had ever known had supported itself by robbing and looting. The Red Army was different. The people were its allies, its kinsfolk. Nothing was to be taken from them, no inconvenience caused them. Regulations governing the conduct of army-men were put to music, to a tune so simple and catchy that every soldier could sing it on the march until it sank deep into his consciousness. And to kill two birds with one stone and learn some Chinese characters at the same time, the marching soldiers would carry boards on their backs with one character from the song written on each board, so that each could learn from the man in front.

Soldiers in the People's Liberation Army no longer need to learn characters in this way, but the spirit of the song is as alive today as when it was first sung and for millions of Chinese it symbolizes those characteristics which make the People's Liberation Army so dear to the people.

Another outstanding impression from my first National Day Parade came right at the end when the marchers had all gone by and the vast Tien An Men square seemed momentarily empty. Then from the back of the square, where they had been patiently waiting for hours, tens of thousands of Young Pioneers rushed forward towards the Gate of Heavenly Peace, towards their beloved leader, releasing doves which circled in the sun-drenched autumn air and a myriad of balloons which soared into the blue canopy of the sky. Rosy cheeked, red-scarved, cheering lustily, full of vigour and happiness, they surged forward like a tidal wave, the rising generation of New China, the generation that would continue the herculean task for which so many millions had sacrificed their lives.

I felt a painful lump in my throat and looking round me I saw tears in many eyes.

I started work a few weeks later.

At first I cycled to the teaching hospital to which I had been appointed, the road taking me over the long marble bridge separating the ancient artificial lakes called respectively the 'North Sea' and 'Middle South Sea'. When the Tibetan style Dagoba in Pei Hai (North Sea) park was wreathed in morning mist the scene was entrancingly beautiful.

By contrast, the hospital was dark and gloomy. It had been the headquarters of the Japanese military intelligence organization and thousands of patriotic Chinese had come to an heroic but painful end within its walls. Hospital beds were crowded close together for this was before large-scale hospital building had started in Peking. Patients' friends and relatives added to the general overcrowding and I felt indignant when a sheep-skin coated peasant hawked noisily and spat on the floor. Thinking to shame him, I fixed him in a disapproving stare and glanced repeatedly at the spittle on the floor. He was puzzled by my disapproval and he too looked down at the floor to see what harm his spit was doing. Certainly my performance did nothing to shame him and looking back on it across the years, I do not feel proud of my own behaviour. Spitting is a bad habit and one day it will go, but I had no right to expect that within five years of Liberation this centuries-old custom would have disappeared. This may well have been the first time that the peasant had ever been inside a building that had anything other than an earthen floor. Spitting must be eliminated but there are many more important things to eliminate first. And the way to set about it is by patient education and not by angrily miming disapproval.

Soon afterwards I witnessed a dramatic success by a traditional Chinese doctor. In accordance with Mao's insistence on the need for doctors of the modern and traditional schools to co-operate with and learn from each other, there were traditional doctors on the staff of every hospital.

I had been consulted about a young woman who was suffering from a dangerous blood disease as a result of which she was bleeding copiously from the gums, bladder and vagina. She had lost a great deal of blood and was in a dangerously anaemic condition. The accepted modern treatment for this condition is an operation to remove the spleen, but in spite of repeated blood transfusions and the use of every drug known to modern medicine, she was thought to be too weak to withstand the operation. My advice was that, since operation was the only thing that could save her life, we would have to run the risk. Accordingly, after a really massive blood transfusion, we operated very speedily while the blood still ran into her vein.

She stood the operation well, but after it, to our dismay, still continued to bleed. When it looked as if there were no hope, the relatives asked us to call in a traditional herbalist doctor.

He stood by the bedside, tall, bearded and dignified, accompanied by his apprentice. Placing her wrist on a velvet cushion, for several minutes he felt first her right and then her left pulse using his index, middle and ring fingers. The apprentice produced a brush and an ink block and the herbalist, after a few moments contemplation, wrote a prescription in beautifully formed characters that covered a whole page. We asked how many doses she should take and were told, 'Only one. We will be back to see her tomorrow. She may need a different medicine then.'

Later I learned that traditional doctors, unlike their modern colleagues, seldom prescribe more than one dose of medicine since they reason, very logically, that if the medicine is effective, the condition will change after the first dose and if it is ineffective, there is no point in continuing with it.

Within twelve hours she stopped bleeding. We were astonished and delighted, but when the old herbalist called again the next day he was not at all surprised and in a matter-of-fact way, prescribed a different medicine to build up her strength.

Within a few weeks she walked out of the hospital, cured and healthy.

Of course, it is possible that it was just a coincidence; that she might have been on the point of recovering when she took the herbalist's medicine. Doubts of this kind are inseparable from every new form of treatment and in fact it is extremely difficult to prove the efficacy of any drug. But my impression is that such cures happen rather too frequently to be explained by coincidence and it is more likely that Chinese herbal remedies may sometimes succeed where modern drugs are ineffective.

In addition to the usual run of recent injuries which I had been accustomed to seeing in England, I also saw many old, neglected cases of which I had no previous experience. They were a legacy from the almost total medical neglect of the labouring people before Liberation. I saw dislocations of the hip, elbow and shoulder which had remained unreduced for ten years and more; fractures that had united in positions of extreme deformity or had not united at all; joints that had become stiff as a result of no treatment or bad treatment; tuberculosis of bones and joints that had been allowed to run riot. I saw patients who had lost limbs years before and had made their own artificial limbs because none were forthcoming from any other source. I saw a youth whose penis had been chopped off by a landlord because his father couldn't pay the rent. I saw a girl from Inner Mongolia who hadn't been able to sit or squat since childhood because of scarring of the buttocks due to a burn.

In the old days, these patients had no hope of getting treatment. Now they could come to Peking from the four corners of the land and they presented a challenge to our little corps of medical workers, lacking in numbers and in skill, who had the responsibility of treating them. As for myself, I was regarded as an expert, but I was seeing such cases for the first time and had less experience of them than those I was supposed to train. I had to go to school all over again, learning from my colleagues and my patients and applying my previous experience to new problems. I was spurred on in this by the urgency and magnitude of the task which confronted us.

I had not been long at work before it became clear that meetings, big and small, played a very important part in the life of the hospital staff. Some were confined to a single ward, others involved everyone in the hospital, from the directors to the laundry workers. We sometimes discussed local matters such as why an operation had failed to achieve the expected result, who should be nominated to attend a conference for model workers, how a complaint by a patient should be dealt with, how we could increase the number of beds without additional staff or additional building, how we could improve the efficiency of the out-patient department, etc., etc. Sometimes we discussed national or international questions such as why agriculture should be regarded as the foundation of the national economy and industry the leading factor, what role the health service could play in supporting agriculture, whether we were satisfied with our Trade Union, why the Chinese government aided newly emerging countries, and whether medical workers could make a contribution to such aid, etc., etc.

At first I was impatient of these incessant meetings which took up much time and interfered with our work. Gradually I understood their value and importance. Many of the problems discussed could have been quickly settled by a decision from above and if this had been done, we might have got through more work. But the policy of the Chinese Communist Party is that, no matter how pressing the immediate tasks may be, long-term interests must always take precedence over short-term interests and unless the persons actually concerned have had an opportunity to debate problems and formulate policy, decisions handed down from above are liable to be wrong. Moreover, unless those who have to operate a policy are convinced of its correctness, it is likely to remain a policy on paper only. In the long run, the key to high working efficiency is to make correct decisions on the basis of unity of purpose, after a detailed examination of all the facts and a full democratic consultation of those involved, and to ensure that everyone understands and supports these decisions.

That is also the style of work of the People's Liberation Army. During the long years of war, before every battle, commanders and men got together to discuss the situation and to work out suitable tactics and strategy. And the more urgent the situation, the more necessary it was considered to hold such discussions.

Facts have proved that this method of work has great advantages.

A problem that I encountered early in the course of my medical work in China was the reluctance of relatives to permit post-mortem examinations or anatomical studies to be carried out on patients who had died. Such examinations are invaluable for checking on the correctness of the diagnosis and treatment and are an important method of raising standards. But age-old beliefs and customs do not disappear overnight and most Chinese are still unwilling to allow the bodies of their dear ones to be dissected.

While on a home visit, I once mentioned this to an old missionary doctor who had taught anatomy in China for several years. He told me that in his time there had been no such problem; the Kuomintang authorities were willing and able to supply an unlimited number of fresh corpses from their concentration camps for Communist suspects. The only trouble was that they had usually been beheaded. When the inconvenience of this was pointed out to a camp commander, he immediately offered to strangle them instead.

A kaleidoscope of street scenes flash back into my mind.

The relaxed and happy people, purposeful but out-going, self-respecting and respecting others, calling each other 'comrade' because they felt like comrades.

The adults dressed in an austere uniformity which led me into many perplexities for I often could not tell if I was talking to a cook or a professor.

Only the babies were really well-dressed with their fur-trimmed bunny-rabbit hats and quilted cloaks of shiny red silk.

The women, for so long oppressed and despised, now showing their new-found freedom in the dignity of their every movement. The old women, with tiny triangular bound feet, better dressed than the others, velvet hats with jade ornaments on their heads, hair tied in a bun, wearing padded trousers even before the weather turned cold.

The children, full of fun, overbrimming with joy. It is rare to see children fight or cry in Peking and even rarer to see them scolded or hit. If a Western child psychologist were to investigate the reasons why juvenile delinquency is so infrequent in China, his inquiries would lead him into areas where he would not expect to venture, for the chief reason is that the ending of exploitation has greatly reduced the social tensions and insecurity which in other societies make themselves felt among all age-groups and provide the soil for juvenile delinquency.

Another reason, not unconnected with the first, is that in sharp contrast both to the despotic parents of feudal China and to the apocryphal Western mother who despatched her husband to 'see what the children are doing and tell them to stop it', modern Chinese parents, in their sane, meaningful society, respect their youngsters and trust them to do the right thing.

They are by no means pampered, but are respected as human beings having their own abilities and desires. I remember travelling on a very crowded bus during the hard years when, due to a succession of natural calamities and other reasons, grain was scarce and eggs were even scarcer. A baby, less than two years of age, was sitting on its mother's lap, hemmed in by tight-packed, swaying standing passengers. The mother shelled a hard-boiled egg and gave it to the baby. His little fingers could hardly grasp the slippery egg and I was fearful that it would fall. But the mother had no such worries. Slowly and carefully the child ate the egg, catching every crumb, until it was all eaten. I think that most Western mothers, who travel in greater comfort and who can buy eggs more easily, would not have trusted the child as much as this Chinese mother did. They would have resisted the child's desire to feed himself and tension would have built up between them.

Chinese children are loved by the whole family, not in a possessive way as flesh and blood of particular parents but as lovable human beings in their own right. Grandparents often do more than parents in bringing up babies, and older children, even those from neighbouring families, also do their share and do it willingly because they want to and it is the normal thing for them to do. When I worked in a leprosy village in the south of China, I loved to watch the nurses come home in the evening from the island in the river where the lepers lived, to the settlement where we all lived together. Before coming home they would have bathed and changed their clothes to avoid the risk of infection. As they came up the path, the babies they had left behind in the care of grannies and grandpas would run towards them, be swept up, kissed and cuddled and passed from hand to hand. The children didn't necessarily run to their own mother but to any mother. And they got the same loving welcome whoever they went to. I often found it difficult to tell which child belonged to which mother. Some so-called experts in the West would deplore the apparent lack of a 'special child-mother relationship' and conclude that this must be 'psychologically traumatizing', but the relationship between children and parents was excellent, the children were happy, co-operative and full of fun and were growing up into thoroughly well-adjusted adults.

On the streets, a complete absence of beggars, vagrants, teddy-boys and prostitutes. In the shops, fixed prices, no persuasion, scrupulous honesty and no bartering. What a contrast with Shanghai 1937!

Road-side stalls roasting chestnuts in mechanically operated cauldrons, filling the air with mouth-watering fragrance. It seemed strange that in China, where so much is done by hand, chestnut roasting should be mechanized.

The variegated traffic. Buses and trams packed until it seemed that they must burst at the seams, clanking and clattering along pot-holed roads. Today, the buses are still tight-packed but they no longer clatter for the roads are smooth and they are mostly trolley buses. As for the trams, they have all but disappeared.

Pedicabs had already replaced the rickshaws of yesteryear and they, too, are now giving way to motorized tricycle taxis.

Donkeys pulling carts laden with great piles of vegetables, hammocks of sacking suspended beneath their buttocks to catch the precious manure and keep the streets clean.

Cars and taxis hooting furiously.

Bicycles galore. It is said that Peking has more bicycles on the roads than any city in the world and those who know say that Chinese-made bicycles are rivalled only by the best British bicycles.

There even used to be camels in the suburbs of Peking, bringing in coal from a mine on the far outskirts. My children used to delight in seeing the camel processions, the young camels, unladen, ambling beside their supercilious elders for training in road sense. I have seen no camels in Peking for many a year.

An old-style funeral at the corner of the lane where we used to live. Everything the deceased could possibly need in the after-life, houses, money, food, servants, horses, cattle and much else had been beautifully made of papier mâché and bamboo, all waiting to be burnt on the day of interment. A tent had been erected where a round-the-clock hot buffet was available for mourners and others. Buddhist monks chanted prayers and played strange and noisy musical instruments. On the last day, the musicians really let themselves go and went in for all kinds of antics such as playing the trumpet through their noses.

Such funeral ceremonies, reeking with superstition and costing so much that the bereaved might be plunged into debt for years, are no longer to be seen in Peking. Now the emphasis is on simplicity and the trend is towards cremation. Grave mounds, which wasted much agricultural land and interfered with ploughing, are, with the descendants' permission, being flattened and the coffins moved to public cemeteries.

Old-style Peking opera, unchanged for centuries, all about emperors, courtesans, long-dead statesmen and ghosts. Gorgeous costumes, stylized acting and singing, librettos so archaic that the incomprehensible words had to be projected on to screens at the side of the stage. The shows went on for hours and the audience's lack of interest was shown by the incessant hum of conversation and cracking of sunflower seeds. And the noise! The singers competed with bands composed largely of gongs and deafening cymbals. I saw my first Peking opera in company with a devotee and at one point, while a singer was trying hard to make himself heard above the din of the orchestra, for no apparent reason the audience suddenly burst into applause. I asked whether it was because he had broken through the sound barrier, but my companion, unamused, replied that it was because he had sung very well.

Old-style opera has now been superseded by operas on modern themes.

The singing, the movements and the quality (though not the quantity) of music are largely unchanged, but the gorgeous costumes have gone and the content is completely transformed. The audiences now are much bigger, more attentive and more enthusiastic than they used to be, for what they now see reflects a life they know, that they themselves are building.

The modernization of Peking opera, like much else, involved a struggle between two lines; between those who clung tenaciously to the past, who wished to glorify long dead despotic rulers, and their hangers-on, who were insensitive to new needs and new thinking, who used the theatre either as a brake on progress or as an escape from reality; and those who understood that for the theatre to flourish it must throw off the shackles of the past, march in step with the people, serve their needs, satisfy their desires, entertain and inspire them.

The parks. Centuries-old pines, propped and supported, their hollow trunks filled like carious teeth cared for by a good dentist. White-skin pines, tall, smooth, and elegant as a lovely woman. Huge ginko trees, dating from the Tang dynasty or earlier, representatives of a nearly extinct species, their leaves fanshaped with no central vein, their fruit much prized by Chinese herbalists. Storytellers holding their audiences entranced. Children's palaces where youngsters can do anything from making plasticine models to running real hydro-electric stations. Halls for chess, for singing, dancing, reciting verse, play acting, making music. Halls for the people. Open air theatres, teashops, fruit stalls. Lakes for boating, swimming, fishing and, in winter, for skating too. Exhibitions for those who like to combine relaxation with edification. On one occasion I entered what I thought was a display of Chilean art to find myself in an exhibition on the cause, spread, consequences and prevention of measles!

The extraordinary honesty of people in New China. I never lock anything up and nothing has ever been missing.

A prominent former Labour MP who visited China told me how he had tried unsuccessfully to get rid of a pair of slippers he didn't want. As he left his hotel in Peking for a tour of China, he put the slippers in the waste-paper basket, but just before the train pulled out of the station, the hotel floor attendant came running along the platform and threw them in through the window. After a day and a night on the train, he wrapped up the slippers and put them under the seat. The next day they turned up at his hotel. He threw them out of his bedroom window but a passer-by picked them up and handed them in. He returned to Peking by air and left them in the car that drove him to the airport. A few days later, they were delivered to his Peking hotel by registered post. Finally he took his slippers back to England.

My first visit to an agricultural co-operative, long before the days of People's Communes. I was shown round by an enthusiastic, voluble old man who turned out to be the animal feeder. He talked non-stop for an hour, telling me of the Co-op's achievements and problems, introducing me to his animals, telling me about their feeding habits. When I asked him if he had been brought up on a farm, his flood of talk came to an abrupt halt and his exuberance evaporated. 'It's funny you should ask that', he said. 'We never lived in any fixed place. All my family except granny and myself died of starvation while

I was still very young. Granny seemed to keep alive on nothing and as for me, until I was eleven or twelve, things weren't too bad for there were a lot of camels where we lived and I used to pick seeds out of their droppings, wash them and eat them. It seems that there are some things that camels can't digest and we can. The trouble was that I had no trousers and when I got bigger it wasn't decent to go out without trousers. I used to borrow granny's trousers when she wasn't using them but she too had to look for food and so we went very hungry.' He paused for a long time. 'Until I joined this Co-operative, I never in my life had known what it felt like to have a full belly.'

The ability of the Chinese to laugh at themselves and recognize their short-comings. I remember, in those early days, going to an industrial exhibition. There were proud rows of shining lathes, diesel engines, turbines, cameras, medical equipment and such like, but one large hall exhibited only faulty products. The centre piece was a string of kettles suspended from the ceiling, each leaky kettle dripping water into the one below. There was a pile of enamel wash-basins, so tightly jammed into each other that a fifty kilogram weight couldn't pull them apart. A shot-gun was on display beneath a cartoon showing a cocky bird on a branch telling a huntsman whose gun had a cork-screw barrel, 'Try again comrade—you'll never hit me with that!' The most telling exhibit was a huge photograph of a young man with a black eye whose grin revealed two missing front teeth. Beneath the photograph was a chest expander with two broken springs.

Enough meandering along the byways of the past, pleasant though I find it to recall the background to the present. I must get on with my main task, which is to sketch those aspects of China's medical services of which I have personal experience, which throw light on the overall political and social development and which help to explain the source of China's dynamism and vitality.

I shall not hesitate to show where there have been clashes between opposing viewpoints and tendencies, for such contradictions nearly always have a political basis and it is precisely in the course of resolving them that progress is made.

Neither shall I avoid entering into the political arena for politics are so dominant in the thinking of the Chinese people, and so directly guide their actions, that any book on present day China that fought shy of discussing political issues would be trivial and one-sided.

I shall not try to write an erudite or comprehensive work on medicine in China. The time is not yet ripe for such a book and when it is, it will need a much wiser author than myself to write it.

4

My teachers—the patients

All doctors learn from their patients. If we did not do so we could never become doctors at all. Book study merely enables us to observe our patients more accurately, to detect changes we might otherwise overlook, and to utilize other doctors' practical experience.

In China, too, I learn clinical medicine from my patients, but in addition, I learn many other things. My patients in socialist China are a living text-book of politics and history. They teach me about the struggles and oppression of the past, about events which led up to the present. They give me glimpses of what the Man of the future will be like. They teach me that human nature is not a fixed, limiting factor to Man's development but that it can change as society changes. They teach me that the world is a fine place to live in and that it will be even better for future generations. They teach me the meaning of endurance and courage, that ideas can generate a mighty material force.

Of the thousands of patients I have treated in China, a few spring to mind.

The lean, brown Tibetan with straggly hair hanging down beneath his seemingly incongruous Western type hat, who hobbled into my consulting room. As he laboriously pulled off his felt boots and showed me his crippled leg he talked incessantly, pointing here and prodding there. He could speak only Tibetan and his companion, a young Tibetan girl, translated what he said into Chinese. The leg was wasted and deformed. There was a deep constricting scar below the knee and ulcers on the heel were running with pus. The toes were twisted and stiffened and he prodded sharply with his finger to indicate that the leg was numb. He lifted his leg to show the scars behind the knee.

He talked and gesticulated as he told his story.

He had been a serf, owned by a Lhasa nobleman. His job when young had been to look after the nobleman's dogs and horses, but his position in society was greatly inferior to that of his charges. They had food and shelter, while he slept in the open and fed on scraps. One night the cold was so bitter that he crept into a kennel and huddled up beside the dog. Comforted by the unaccustomed warmth he slept soundly and when his master arrived at the stables for an early morning ride, he was still dozing blissfully beside the dog. The nobleman, infuriated that a contemptible serf should soil his fine dog, lashed out wildly. The sleeping youth made the fatal mistake of trying to run away. The punishment for a serf who ran away was hamstringing. It had been so in Tibet since time immemorial, and as soon as the serf was caught, his master drew his dagger and proceeded to inflict the punishment with his own hands. He slashed the tendons behind the knee to make sure the youth would never run away again. Unfortunately for the lad, he slashed not only the tendons but also the nerves so that his leg became permanently paralysed. The wound bled profusely and, to staunch the haemorrhage, the nobleman ordered boiling butter to be poured into the wound. For good measure he chained his victim to a post so tightly that the skin below the knee sloughed away.

Slowly the wounds healed but the leg remained paralyzed. The foot became progressively more deformed and walking barefoot over stony paths caused chronic ulceration of his anaesthetic heel.

In 1959, after the revolt of the Tibetan nobles was crushed, the serfs were freed and democratic reforms instituted. Tibet joined the rest of China on the long road out of the past and into the future.

The crippled ex-serf learned to read and write. He—who had been less than a dog—became a local leader and was elected County head. He consulted the doctors in the newly established hospital in Lhasa, and they advised him to go to Peking.

And so he had come, travelling thousands of miles across mountains and deserts with all expenses paid by the Government.

He indicated that in his opinion it would be best to cut the leg off and give him an artificial one.

His interpreter's voice became choked and she stopped translating. I looked up and saw her eyes were brimming with tears. 'I'm sorry', she said, 'I know it's silly of me to cry—I shouldn't do so. I've heard his story many times and I should be used to it by now. But he's such a good man—and those beasts were so vicious—so brutal. . . .'

The leper in the South of China whose fingers and toes had rotted away. In the sweltering heat, I was selecting suitable patients for surgical treatment. He refused to sit on the offered chair but squatted cross-legged on the earthen floor and with intense concentration and effort started to undo the laces of his canvas shoes. Without fingers it was extremely difficult for him to do so, but, almost angrily, he refused help. The sweat streamed down his face. He held the laces between his fists—he used his teeth. Eventually he removed his shoes and began to unwind the bandages. He would not be helped. He begged my forgiveness for taking up so much time saying it was really a simple job, and he had to do it himself.

At first I felt impatient and then I understood. Disease had eroded his body but not his will. His hands had lost their skill but he was determined not to become dependent on others.

So we waited while he unwound the bandages. When the task was done he wiped his brow with his sleeve and looked up with a little smile of triumph. 'Comrade Doctor—I'm sorry I kept you waiting. I know you must be busy. But it is not pleasant for others to touch my feet.'

In the cool of the evening, I walked along the riverside. The lights of the leprosy hospital were reflected in the water. A water buffalo grazed alongside the sugar-cane. The air was heavy with scents of the night.

Suddenly the sound of singing rang across the river. It was a song of the Chinese revolution. Curious to know who was singing I punted across the water. The same patient was conducting a choir of his fellow lepers, leading the singing in a fine tenor voice.

When the song was finished I asked the leper if music had been his hobby. 'No—it was never my hobby. But we know that all the people are singing songs of the revolution and though we here are physically isolated, in spirit we feel a great unity with all the other people. So we, too, like to sing such songs. You see, Comrade Doctor, you couldn't know what it was like for lepers in the old days. The Japanese had a simple way with people like us—they shot lepers and threw their bodies into the lakes and rivers. The Kuomintang bandits sometimes did the same. Sometimes they just drove us up into the mountains where we starved or froze to death. . . . Now we are cared for, and doctors come from far away to help us. Now we have hope, we can see the way ahead. That is why we like to sing songs of the revolution.'

As I went back across the river, the sound of song followed me on the sweet night air. The lepers were expressing their oneness with their fellow men.

The fourteen year old peasant girl in Shansi province whose leg had been burned to the bone.

Unexpectedly a message had come asking if I was prepared to leave Peking at once to see a patient. Half an hour later, feeling flattered and self-important, I was being driven to a military airfield. The machine was waiting, its engines already warmed up. Two other surgeons were at the airport. We were to fly together. None of us knew our destination—or what kind of patient we were going to see. But we assumed that it must be someone important.

The aircraft flew in a westerly direction. We shared sandwiches with the pilot in complete informality. We landed at Taiyuan airport and were driven to a military hospital. It looked as though we were indeed going to treat a VIP. But the VIP turned out to be not a high-ranking officer or a statesman but the fourteen year old daughter of a peasant.

Nearly two weeks earlier, in rescuing a shepherd and two hundred sheep from death by burning, she had sustained serious burns.

In bitterly cold weather the shepherd had driven his flock into a barn for warmth and shelter. Lambing had just finished, and the young lambs were suffering acutely from the cold. To warm his charges the shepherd lit a charcoal stove but, unfortunately, he was overcome by fumes and fell unconscious, overturning the stove. The dry timbers of the barn caught alight and the fire spread rapidly.

Just then the girl passed, on her way home from school. She heard the bleating of the terrified sheep, and the crackle of flames. She tried to open the door, but the shepherd had bolted it on the inside.

Unhesitatingly she climbed a drainpipe, smashed the glass skylight, and dropped twenty feet into the inferno. Although she had broken her ankle in landing, she forced the door open, dragged out the unconscious shepherd, drove the terrified sheep through the flames to safety and finally rolled on the shepherd to extinguish his still-smouldering padded clothes.

By the time help arrived, she herself had been badly burnt. She was taken to a military hospital since it was nearby, well equipped and well staffed. Military hospitals often admit civilians, for the revolutionary army has a long tradition of being closely united with the masses of the people. From the time the Red Army first came into being, its relationship with the people in the words of Mao Tse-tung, was the relationship of fish to water.

Now that the People's Liberation Army is a mighty military force, as a matter of basic policy it unites even more closely with the masses of the people.

The girl's early treatment had been excellent. The fracture of the right ankle had been set and immobilized and shock from the extensive burns had been prevented by scientifically controlled intravenous infusions of blood and plasma. Infection had been controlled by occlusive dressings, by strict isolation and by the use of antibiotics.

But the burn was exceptionally deep and by the fourteenth day after burning, a dangerous and perplexing condition had developed. The main part of the burn involved the left leg from just above the ankle up to the buttocks and waist. All the skin here had sloughed away revealing burnt muscle and bone. The burn was deepest around the knee joint where the charred bone and the interior of the joint was exposed. All the tendons and ligaments crossing the knee had been destroyed and the only intact structures connecting the thigh to the lower leg were the main blood vessels and nerves. These, miraculously, still functioned but they could be seen to twist and bend with every movement.

That was where the danger lay and it was to discuss how best to handle this problem that we had been called in from Peking. If the artery, surrounded by sloughing and infected tissues, continued to be twisted and bent, it would almost certainly rupture and a fatal haemorrhage might result. Even if it did not rupture, the blood inside it would probably clot, causing gangrene of the limb.

With our military medical colleagues, and the junior doctors and nurses treating the girl, we discussed the problem far into the night. Finally, we settled on a course of action. We were able to agree because we all approached the problem from the common standpoint of wanting to do the best we could for the heroic young girl. We tried hard to put aside all considerations of prestige, or seniority, to be modest and open-minded and to be willing to be convinced by others' arguments.

Some were in favour of amputating through the thigh, because this would eliminate the danger of haemorrhage and reduce the duration of the illness. Others argued that this would expose clean tissues to the danger of infection, that no skin was available to cover the stump, and such an operation might be followed by septicaemia.

To overcome these disadvantages, others favoured amputating through the knee joint for the knee joint was already infected and since the lower leg was attached only by its nerves and blood vessels, the operation would be simple and safe. But some were against any kind of amputation because, miraculously, the foot still had normal blood supply, nerve supply and skin. Although the patient was in danger, her condition was by no means desperate. Even if the artery ruptured, provided everyone was prepared, it would be possible to stop the haemorrhage within seconds.

Eventually we decided to try and save the limb.

The next problem was to work out a method for achieving our objective. The main risk arose from uncontrolled movements at the knee joint for these constantly endangered the main artery. But to eliminate these movements was extremely difficult. We could not use external splintage or a plaster cast since the skin and underlying soft tissue had been destroyed right up to the waist.

We decided on a bold plan. Even though the surface of the bone had been burnt, its deeper parts must be still living. If we sliced off the cartilage-covered surfaces of the bones forming the knee joint and clamped the raw surfaces tightly together, they should unite even though there was infection and even though the rim of the bone was dead. If this succeeded, the danger to the blood vessels would be eliminated and later on we could remove the dead bone around the rim and apply skin grafts directly to the healthy bone. The function of the knee joint would of course be lost, but this was inevitable whatever we did. Our aim was to get a soundly healed limb with a stiff knee, a good hip, a good foot and a normal blood supply and nerve supply.

The next day we operated and everything turned out as planned. Within six weeks the bones had grown together and the whole limb had been covered with skin grafts. Two weeks later she began walking and was transferred to a lakeside sanatorium for convalescence.

Some years later, accompanied by the shepherd whose life she had saved, she came to see me in Peking. She said that her leg gave her no trouble and that she was able to work just like the other commune members. But the shepherd said that she was being modest, that in fact she worked outstandingly well and had been elected a model worker three years in succession.

She said that if it had not been for the solicitude shown by the Party after she had burned her leg, she would not have been able to work at all and probably would not have survived.

Remembering the care lavished on her, the special aircraft, the hours of debate, the isolation suite in the hospital, and the twenty-four hours a day nursing, I was inclined to agree with her. In New China the common people are the VIPs, and nothing is too good for them.

The girl with the smiling eyes and flying pigtails whom I first knew as a train attendant, and later as a patient.

She served tea and brought sunshine into the carriage as our train rumbled through the snow-covered countryside. We chatted about this and that until my companion, something of an expert in Chinese dialects, asked her where she came from. She named the area and my companion said, 'I thought so. During the Anti-Japanese war, I lived in a village in that county for many months. I had been wounded and thought I was finished. A peasant woman took me into her house and nursed me back to health. At that time the Japanese were operating their "Three All" policy—"kill all, burn all, loot all". But this village had worked out an answer. The people had built an ingenious system of tunnels, which honeycombed the area and not only provided a refuge for the villagers, but also enabled them to strike back at their tormentors. Side-tunnels branched off from the main system, and one of them came to the surface in the house where I had found refuge. Whenever the Japanese came, she would carry me down into the tunnel, for I was too weak to walk. She was a wonderful woman. Her husband had been killed and she was left with three children, the youngest just a little baby. But she kept the family together and fearlessly helped our Red Army men.'

As my companion reminisced, the pigtails stopped flying and the smiling eyes misted over. 'I wonder if it's possible,' she asked him. 'Could you possibly be Uncle Gao who used to play with me and make me wooden whistles? That Uncle Gao had a beard and was very thin.'

My companion, excited, gripped her hand and looked into her face. He whispered, 'Where were you born? What is your surname?' She replied, 'I was born in Chen Family village—my surname is Chen. My mother was eventually caught by the Japanese.'

For the next two days our train chugged through frozen country and the girl train attendant frequently came to see us. She was, indeed, the daughter of the peasant woman who had saved my companion's life.

I noticed that she limped and had a deformed foot. I asked her to see me in Peking, so that we could get an X-ray and make a thorough examination. A few weeks later she arrived. The foot had been dislocated for many years and the tendons and bones had become moulded in the dislocated position. When I asked her how it had happened, her smiling eyes again clouded over with sadness.

'It was so long ago, I hardly remember. And yet I can never completely forget. Not long after Uncle Gao had left us to rejoin his Army unit, the Japanese unexpectedly arrived in our village. All who could went down into the tunnels, but my mother had the children to look after and she had time only to get two of us into the tunnel when she heard the Japanese nearby. To make sure they wouldn't find the entrance to the tunnel, she quickly covered it up, and ran out of the house towards the forest, with me on her shoulders. It was night time and she gripped my feet tight so that I shouldn't fall off. We had nearly reached the forest when a Japanese soldier saw us and shot my mother. As she fell she seemed to grip my feet even tighter. That is when my foot must have been dislocated for it has never been right since then.

'My foot doesn't really matter, Comrade Doctor. I just limp a little and occasionally it aches. In a way, it's even a good thing because it reminds me of my mother and father and all the other comrades who suffered so much to free our land. And that makes me determined to work and study better as a way of repaying the debt I owe them.'

The smile had returned to her eyes.

The two girl students from Peking University. So different and yet so alike.

Cheng, slim, delicate and graceful, the only daughter of a family of intellectuals. Made much of by her brother. Never knowing want or hardship.

Wu, from a poor peasant family. Tall, heavily built, with a finely chiselled face. Long before she reached maturity she had known cold, pain and hunger for she had been sold as a child bride.

In the old days it would have been said that they had been born under different stars. But they grew up under the same star—under China's five-pointed red star. This united them more than their different social backgrounds separated them. They shared the enthusiasm, the patriotism, the sense of dedication which is characteristic of modern Chinese youth.

From their first day in the faculty of chemistry, they had been good friends. They argued fiercely but their arguments cemented their friendship. Cheng was a great success in the social life of the college. She sang like a lark and danced with fire and grace. Wu was more stolid. She studied diligently, assiduously helped her fellow students, was athletic and won a place in the college basketball team. Both of them joined the Young Communist League, and both were elected model students.

During the tempestuous year of the Big Leap Forward, factories became colleges and colleges became factories. They were years of experimentation, of innovation, of releasing a torrent of long pent-up creative initiative. Students in grade three of the faculty of chemistry combined their studies with the production of pure ether, needed in large quantities for a multitude of experiments, and Wu and Cheng threw themselves whole-heartedly into the work.

One day a bottle of ether in the laboratory caught fire. On the same bench were nine stills, all distilling ether and nearby shelves were loaded with corrosive and inflammable chemical reagents. If the bottle of ether were to explode, the laboratory would be ablaze in a few moments, the whole building might be destroyed and loss of life might be heavy.

Cheng grabbed the bottle of flaming ether and raced for the door. But Wu was there before her. She snatched the bottle from Cheng's hands and ran downstairs and out into the courtyard. By this time the bottle had become a mass of flames which splashed over Wu's face, hands and clothes. She hurled the bottle away just as Cheng appeared carrying a blazing still which exploded in her hands, drenching her in flames and knocking her to the ground. Without a moment's hesitation, Wu carried her to safety and with bare hands ripped off her blazing clothes. Wu herself became a ball of fire.

The force of the explosion shattered window panes and leaping flames threatened to engulf the building. The other students formed a human wall and beat back the flames.

Within half an hour I was helping to treat the girls in our emergency department.

There had not yet been time for shock to develop and both girls were mentally alert. Their faces and hands were charred and dry, the hair, eyebrows and eyelashes had been burnt away. Blisters were starting to form on their bodies, a warning that shock would not be long in developing unless active preventive measures were taken.

Within minutes we had plasma infusions running into their veins at a rate guided by half-hourly checks on the blood pressure, the amount of urine and the degree of blood concentration.

The girls lay on adjacent couches in the shock room. Speaking was difficult since their lips were stiffened and hot gases had scorched their throats. Nevertheless they comforted each other, each insisting that the other be treated first, both asking about the laboratory and their fellow students.

Gradually the drugs we had given them took effect and they became drowsy. When we were sure that our anti-shock measures were effective, we removed them to separate isolation rooms where we cleansed and dressed the burns.

They remained in their separate rooms, isolated from the outside world, for many weeks. But although they were isolated, their conduct during their long ordeal was an unending inspiration and a profound education to other patients in the Burns block, to the ten thousand students in Peking University and, above all, to the nurses, doctors, orderlies, dieticians, and laboratory workers who looked after them.

They communicated with each other by writing notes, sometimes three or four times a day. They themselves couldn't write for their hands had been burnt, but they whispered their messages to a nurse who acted as scribe and postman.

'My dear comrade,' wrote Wu, 'I can see how thin I am getting even though most of my body is bandaged up. You must be getting thin too, and you were always much slimmer than I. The doctors urge me to eat more. They tell me that I need plenty of protein food at this stage. I know they are right but I find it awfully difficult to eat. I'm just not in the slightest bit hungry. I know it must be the same with you. So let's have a competition to see who can be the biggest glutton. Today for lunch I will eat three eggs, two ounces of rice and drink a big glass of milk. Even though I hate milk I will do it. Tell me what you will eat.'

And Cheng replied, 'Dearest sister—I accept your challenge. Today for lunch I ate a huge meat ball with my rice and then, like you, I drank milk and finally I had an orange. You too should eat oranges. I am getting better quickly and my eyes are unharmed. The nurse tells me that your eyes too were not scorched by the flames, but maybe she is just saying that to console me. Please tell me yourself—are your eyes quite normal? I'll believe what you say because I know how strong and principled you are.'

Hundreds of notes passed between them, full of encouragement, courage and mutual love.

A deputation of students came to visit them. They were not allowed into the ward because of the risk of cross-infection but they and the patients could see each other through the glass partition. They were warned not to allow their expressions to convey their horror at what they saw and after signalling their greetings, they sent in the gifts and letters they had brought. Students from the Fine Art faculty had painted a picture of Chairman Mao for each of them. The music department sent them a specially composed song. The college gardeners sent masses of flowers, fruit and fine vegetables. Their class-mates sent them a volume of poems by Mao Tse-tung.

When the visitors left, they took with them the charred remains of the girls' clothing.

Later, on the college campus, 10,000 students assembled to hear a report from the deputation and to receive into safe keeping the scorched clothing. As it was being handed over, something firm was felt in a pocket. It was a pocket edition of Mao Tse-tung's article, 'Serve the People'. Though the print was scarcely legible, marginal notes and comments could still be made out.

The students, many of them moved to tears, left that meeting determined to become worthy school-mates of Wu and Cheng.

As the dead skin sloughed away, the raw areas were skin grafted under local anaesthesia. Though the operations were painful, both girls refused drugs because they made them drowsy and interfered with the study programme which they had decided on and rigidly adhered to. While her hands were bandaged, Wu had worked out a method of turning the pages with a chopstick held in her teeth. Cheng improved it by attaching pieces of rubber to both ends of the chopstick. They wanted to ease the burden on the busy nurses who, for their part, considered it a privilege to help them in any way they could.

Mainly they studied the writings of Chairman Mao and many of the notes which passed between them were about some passage in Mao's works.

Gradually their wounds healed and the great day came when the two friends, their friendship enriched by the long travail which they had endured in common, could be together.

Their faces were hideously distorted and before they were allowed to see each other the doctors and nurses discussed how to arrange things so as to lessen the shock, for neither of the girls had seen a mirror. In the end we decided that there was really nothing we could do. When they saw each other for the first time they stood still, looked at each other for the briefest moment and then threw their arms round each other.

Wu laughed. 'My! You do look a sight! But I'm sure I look much worse since I was never as pretty as you.'

'Let's get a mirror,' said Cheng, 'and face up to the facts. We should be a hit as the Ugly Sisters in college dramatics even if there's no other part for us.'

The doctors explained that plastic surgery could improve their appearance, but they were not greatly interested. 'We've had enough surgery for the time being,' they said. 'First get our hands supple again and then let's talk about our faces.'

So we started a course of physiotherapy and the function of their hands gradually improved. They argued, correctly, that the best therapy was actual work and so they did nursing and cleaning work in the wards, scrubbing the floors, serving meals, feeding patients, and reading and writing for patients who requested it. In the children's ward, they told the children stories and helped those of school age to make up the lessons they were missing.

One day they decided to amuse the children with a song and dance which they had composed themselves. While they were performing, a tiny tot who had just been admitted to hospital, shut his eyes tightly and called out, 'Stop singing—stop dancing—you are ugly.'

An older child put his arms around the tiny tot and said to him, 'Open your eyes, little brother. Look at them. They are not ugly. They are beautiful.'

5

Three-legged donkey

Old Zhang had been a good patient. His pelvic bone had been splintered and the main ligament on the inner side of the knee ruptured by a fall of rock while excavating a water-cistern two months before. The pelvic fracture had caused blood to collect under the skin of the buttock and this gave rise to a problem in treatment, for while it was necessary to relieve pressure on the buttock in order to prevent sloughing of the skin, the best method of treatment for the knee injury required him to lie flat on his back.

We tackled this problem by driving screws into the prominent part of the hip bone on each side and attaching a system of weights and pulleys to them to lift the buttocks clear of the bed, thus relieving the skin of all pressure. Then, with a needle and syringe we aspirated the collection of blood and injected an enzyme to help the absorption of any that remained.

The pelvic injury must have bruised the nerves to the bladder for the patient was unable to pass urine. To deal with this we called in a colleague from the acupuncture department. The Chinese traditional doctor, bearded and dignified, felt the pulse, nodded sagely and in a completely matter-of-fact way, told the patient that his problem would be solved immediately. This unbounded confidence in the efficacy of their treatment is characteristic of traditional doctors and probably contributes not a little to their success. He cleaned the skin with alcohol and iodine and, with a delicate twirling motion, inserted fine acupuncture needles into the chosen spots. Within a few minutes the patient was able to pass urine and from that time onward he had no further bladder trouble.

There were three possible lines of treatment for the ruptured knee ligament and we debated the merits and demerits of each of them. One method was to immobilize the whole lower limb in a plaster cast until the ligament had healed. This method was simple but it had the disadvantage that as the swelling subsided, the plaster cast would become loose and the ligament might heal with the knee in a slightly knock-kneed position. Moreover, immobilization causes muscle wasting and joint stiffness which delays full recovery. Another method was to operate on the knee to stitch the torn ends of the ligament together. This could ensure normal healing of the ligament, but every operation is associated with a certain risk and many of us thought that if the same result could be obtained without operating, then it was better not to do so.

The method that we finally decided to use combined the principles of Chinese traditional medicine and modern surgery. Chinese traditional doctors believe that controlled movements do not interfere with the healing of torn tissues or broken bones but, on the contrary, promote healing. We therefore neither immobilized the knee nor operated on it, but used a method of splinting which guaranteed that knock-knee deformity could not develop and which permitted the patient to exercise the knee while the ligament was healing.

Within a week, when all danger of sloughing of the skin of the buttock had passed, we removed the screws and allowed him to lie normally in bed. Soon afterwards he was able to bend the knee to a right-angle and to straighten it without help. Since he came from a mountainous region, and needed strong legs, we next concentrated on re-developing muscle power. We tied a sandbag to his ankle when he exercised, so that he had to contract his muscles more powerfully and Old Zhang, determined to recover as quickly and as completely as possible, constantly urged us to increase the weight of the sandbag.

I often visited Old Zhang in the ward for he was a racy conversationalist and I enjoyed his reminiscences and his descriptions of his present life. Like 500 million other Chinese peasants, he was a member of a People's Commune and although, judging from his description, the area where he lived was singularly barren, his enthusiasm for it was unbounded. He often suggested that I should visit him and one day, shortly before he was due to go home, he suddenly became very serious, took hold of my hand and said, 'You know, Comrade Doctor, I'm not just inviting you to visit us out of politeness. I really want you to come. It's true that Peking is the capital, but wonderful things are going on in other parts too. It would be good for you to visit us— even to stay with us for a week or two if you don't mind rough living.' I promised I'd go.

The day before he left the hospital he asked for a bucket of earth from the hospital garden to take back to his Commune. 'You see,' he explained, 'you have plenty of good earth here, but we live in a place where earth is so scarce that whenever any of us goes to a place where soil is plentiful, we bring a little back with us. When you come, Comrade Doctor, perhaps you would also bring some. We'd appreciate it.'

A few weeks later he wrote asking me to visit him the following Sunday.

Old Zhang thanked me for the earth I had brought from Peking, ran his fingers through it appreciatively and sprinkled it on one of the newly-built terraces.

I already knew much of his past, but as we trudged round the village he filled in the details. He had come here thirty-three years ago when he was twenty-one years of age. No one came after him until the Commune was formed in 1958 for there was nothing to come to. The area which he had left had rich soil, but, in good years and bad, the landlord had exploited his family mercilessly until they lost their land and all their possessions. Zhang's mother died and his father joined the flood of landless beggars which streamed over the land. Zhang himself, full of the confidence of youth, went his own way.

After months of wandering he came to the mountains of eastern Hopei province and there, far from warlords and officials, he found shelter with a family as poor and dogged as his own. They never ate grain but lived on flour made from wild Chinese dates, on leaves and wild vegetables.

Even here, the land was owned by a landlord. Zhang visited him in his spacious residence down in the valley and told him that he wished to settle in the mountains, marry and raise a family. 'Certainly, young man. Choose your own mountainside, wherever you like, grow what you like. Build yourself a house. Find a good wife. We need people like you in these parts— young and strong and not afraid of work. You'll do well here—mark my words.' Zhang had a bitter experience of landlords and was not entirely reassured. He explained that he had no money and could pay no rent. 'Rent! Don't think about rent! Just open up the land and raise crops and not until the crops are standing in the fields will I ask you for rent. And even then I won't want much. Just give me sixty pounds of grain a year for every mu you cultivate and I'll be satisfied.' (One mu is one sixth of an acre.)

So Zhang selected a slope and set to work. The whole place was a desert of stones—enough to deter the most lion-hearted of men. No speck of soil was visible on the surface but beneath the stones there was a thin layer. He used some of the stones to make himself a shelter where he slept, and with the others he built low walls so that when the rain fell it would not wash the soil down into the valley.

Before dawn every day he left his shelter and walked ten miles to the county town where he hired himself out as a labourer. In the evenings he continued clearing the land and after a year of back-breaking toil he had cleared and levelled one sixth of an acre. On his way to and from work he collected manure for his plot of earth. When the spring came he planted the land to millet, and now all his energy had to go into carrying water for the precious green shoots.

In the autumn he harvested eighty-five pounds of golden millet—sixty pounds of which he poured into the landlord's granary.

Zhang married a strong, wholesome girl with unbound feet. Between them they enlarged the stone shelter, built a stove and a kang and made a door of millet stalks. Between them they cleared and terraced another mu of land. Zhang made some primitive wooden farming tools, a bucket and a carrying pole.

A son was born. This meant more work for Zhang since his wife could not do as much heavy work as formerly. In good years Zhang could raise enough grain to pay his rent and leave a small surplus. But in 1941, disaster struck. The baby fell ill and nearly all Zhang's savings went in buying herbal remedies. Then the spring rains failed to materialize and the soil became parched and powdery and was scattered by the wind. Zhang trudged endlessly down to the valley for water. One day he found a barricade around the spring in the valley and the landlord's bailiff was standing there demanding payment for each bucket of water. He said that the spring belonged to the landlord and although the landlord was a very kind man and had let the people use it free of charge, he couldn't go on doing this for ever. Zhang felt a surge of desperate anger and asked to see the landlord's title deeds. But the bailiff laughed contemptuously and told him that an illiterate lout like himself couldn't read the title deeds even if he showed them to him.

That autumn Zhang harvested just enough grain to pay his rent. There was no surplus at all. Next year the spring drought was even worse, and in the summer the sparse, spindly millet was battered by downpours of rain which swept away the walls and washed the soil down the mountain side. Zhang, weak from a diet of wild plants, scarcely had the energy to repair the walls of his terraces. He took all his harvest to the landlord but it fell short of the agreed amount by seventy pounds.

The landlord was magnanimous. He didn't beat Zhang or throw him into prison or seize his land. He told him that if his baby had been a girl he might have accepted her in place of the grain for a girl was always useful in the house and one day she would bring in a little dowry. As things were, he was prepared to let Zhang carry forward his debt to the following year, adding an additional seventy pounds by way of interest—providing that Zhang agreed to work on the landlord's land for two days each week until the debt was repaid.

But things didn't work out that way. In 1943, a detachment of the Communist Eighth Route Army occupied Zhang's village. The landlord fled and the villagers ceremoniously burnt all his title deeds. Under the guidance of the Communists, they elected a committee, including Zhang, to look after their affairs. They organized a militia to defend the village and to help the Communist Army in its fight against the Japanese. They set up a school and Zhang, who had never had a day's schooling in his life, laboriously started to learn to read.

Ten years went by. Landlordism, foreign invaders and indebtedness had disappeared from the face of China. Tens of millions of formerly landless peasants had become smallholders. But things couldn't stop there. The peasants were secure in their land tenure but they were still at the mercy of nature.

To move China forward from the past to the future, it was necessary to change individual farming into collective farming. Zhang, by now a seasoned fighter for socialism, saw this need and explained it to his fellow villagers. In 1953, twenty-three of his poor fellow peasants organized themselves into a farming co-operative which the rich peasants sneeringly called the Paupers Co-op.

The Co-op's only draught animal was a donkey which had broken a fetlock some years before. The bones had joined but it still hobbled about on three legs and the Co-op members, as a riposte to the sneering name given by the rich peasants, named their Co-op the Three-Legged Donkey Co-op. Its membership and resources grew rapidly and during the next few years it became well known by this name.

The urgent need was to open up more land for cultivation and to ensure a water supply. The task was huge and the Co-op lacked manpower, money and machinery. They had, however, as Zhang explained to me, one asset which was to prove decisive and this was an unshakeable conviction that by hard work and by relying on their own efforts, they would be able to overcome all difficulties. I asked Zhang what was the source of this inner strength and he replied that it came from the teachings of Mao Tse-tung.

One of Chairman Mao's best known articles is called 'The Foolish Old Man Who Removed the Mountains'. It was delivered as a speech in 1945 at a time when the Communists faced great difficulties, and its purpose was to inspire confidence to overcome these difficulties. It tells of an old man in ancient times whose house faced south but whose view was obstructed by two great mountains. Together with his sons he began to dig away the mountains. A greybeard with a reputation for wisdom saw them doing this and laughed at them for attempting the impossible. But the old man was not daunted and he replied: 'When I die, my sons will carry on; when they die there will be my grandsons and then their sons and grandsons and so on to infinity. High as they are, the mountains can never grow any higher. Every bit that we dig away will make them that much lower. Why can't we clear them away?'

The conviction that by determination and tenacity they could overcome all obstacles gripped the minds of the peasants in the Three-Legged Donkey Co-op and generated in them a force which finally enabled them to transform the barren mountains into fertile terraces. To do this it was not enough just to remove the surface stones, for on most of the slopes there was no soil beneath them. They had to carry the soil, basketful by basketful, from three-quarters of a mile away, and each mu of land needed a minimum of 2,000 baskets of earth. To find water all able-bodied peasants contributed from ten to twenty days of voluntary labour a year to the collective. In fourteen years, 90,000 work days were used in the search for water by a population which never exceeded its present level of 598. The older and more superstitious peasants insisted on asking a geomancer where to dig for water, but after months of fruitless digging they threw superstition to the winds and called in a geologist who located water on the far side of the hill. Here they dug a well, installed an electric pump and laid a pipe over the hill to a cistern twelve yards deep and seventeen yards in diameter which they had hewn out of solid rock. It was while working on this cistern, a key part of the new irrigation system, that Old Zhang had been injured.

In 1958 the Co-op amalgamated with neighbouring Co-ops to become a production brigade in a People's Commune, and from being grain-deficient in 1953, by 1964 they had an average per mu yield of 614 pounds and were able to sell 91,600 pounds to the state.

The thin mountain air parched my lips and the sun reflected from the stone-clad mountain sides dazzled my eyes. For all his recent injury and for all his fifty years of hard toil, Old Zhang, deeply suntanned and sprouting a stubbly little beard, was as nimble as a mountain goat and I had difficulty in keeping up with him. He could see that I was getting tired and suggested that we go down to the village for lunch. On the way down he pointed out landmarks in the village below.

'See those houses with tiled roofs down there?' he said. 'We built those last year. They may not look very grand to you since you come from London, one of the great cities of the world. But we like them very much. The heavy roofs keep out the summer heat and the winter cold. During the past twelve years we have built an extra four rooms per family.

'That building over there is our new school. In the old days the likes of us never had the faintest possibility of going to school—not even to see what it was like. I know, because when I was a kid I was terribly curious to see what went on in school and one day I smuggled myself in. But they found me and kicked me out. They told me I was a disgrace because I had brought fleas into the school.

'Now all the children in the Commune aged eight and over go to school. If a child is sick for any length of time, we have a special teacher who goes to his home to teach him there. This brigade has two primary schools and one half work/half study middle school. We even have four students in University, including my eldest boy who is studying geology in Changsha. When they come home during the vacations they work in the fields with the rest of us.'

We visited the clinic in a brick-walled whitewashed cottage. Members of a mobile medical team were carrying out a health check on the children and were vaccinating youngsters against infantile paralysis. They visited this village every ten days from their headquarters fifteen miles away, making the journey on donkeys. I asked the doctor if he was ever called out to an emergency and he told me that two months before he had performed an operation for obstructed childbirth in the very room where we were talking. He saw me glance at the beaten earth floor and the coarse wooden furniture and said, 'I know what you are thinking. It's true that conditions here are not nearly as good as we would like them to be. But until last year, no doctor or nurse had ever come to this village. Soon there will be enough money to build a much better place—maybe even with tiled walls and running water! But for the time being we have to make do with what we've got. When they called me out two months ago, the peasants scrubbed this place until it was as clean as a new pin. Both mother and baby did very well and there was no infection of the wound.'

He had performed quite a number of operations for obstructed labour because, owing to widespread poverty and malnutrition in the past, rickets had been common and many women had grown up with deformities of the pelvis which prevented natural childbirth.

As we left the clinic a group of strapping girls passed by. 'What do you think of our tough lasses?' Zhang asked. 'No rickets or semistarvation now! That group goes in for tree planting on the highest slopes and is always breaking records. We have planted 102,000 walnut and apple trees, and we plan to plant one million trees during the next three years. Some of our members objected to using so much labour power on tree planting. They said that trees grow slowly and that we should concentrate on quick returns. Others argued that New China is here to stay and we ought to think not only of our own good but also of the coming generations. We argued about this for a long time and in the end everyone agreed to go ahead with tree planting.'

We briefly visited the lame donkey which had inspired the poor peasants' name for their original Co-op. Too old to work, it was comfortably pensioned off and earned its corn by helping to remind the youth that their present good life had been hard won.

Then, to my relief, we reached the cottage where we were to have lunch. We sat on the kang, and chatted with the lean young peasant who was our host as we ate millet porridge, wheaten pancakes and eggs. 'I was born in this village,' he said. 'I was just a nipper when Old Zhang came here. As soon as I was old enough, just like all the other lads, I wanted to leave. The trouble was that there was no better place to go to. Everywhere was just as bad. My old granny persuaded me to stay. Somehow she seemed to know that things would change one day. How right she was! I love this place now and will never leave it. My sweat—and the sweat of my mates—is on every bit of earth and every stone. It's something that we made ourselves out of nothing. Something useful, something beautiful, something that will last for ever. That gives you a fine feeling of contentment.'

An old peasant, with a week's growth of stubble on his chin, came into the cottage. 'Sit down, uncle,' said our host, 'I'm glad you've come. Tell our guest here about your pig. He'll be interested.' He turned to me. 'His name is Wang Chen and he and his pig have become quite famous in these parts.'

Old Wang looked embarrassed. 'Why should he be interested in that defile-mother pig? I wish I'd never set eyes on the animal!'

'He raised that pig from litter,' said our host, 'and it turned out to be an exceptionally clever animal. Some people think pigs are stupid, but they're not. This one followed Old Wang round like a dog. He could find his way home from anywhere. Last New Year's day, Old Wang sold the pig in a market fifteen miles away, and, believe it or not, by the following evening the pig turned up again, his trotters a bit sore but otherwise none the worse. And what's even more remarkable, a couple of days later Old Wang took a full day off work, went back to the market with his faithful pig, found the couple who had bought it from him and returned it to them. You see, Old Wang, if he'll forgive me for saying so, has a reputation for being rather tight-fisted and everyone was amazed that he should give up the pig so readily.'

'You're wrong on two counts,' said Old Wang testily. 'In the first place, I'm not tight-fisted—I'm just careful. If I hadn't been careful I wouldn't have been able to keep alive as long as I have. In the second place, it wasn't easy to give up that pig. My old woman heard him snorting and grunting outside and when she opened the door and he came trotting in, we looked at each other with exactly the same thought in our heads. We'd sold the pig once and now we could sell it again! Believe me, it wasn't easy to decide to return that pig to its rightful owner. My wife and I talked it over half the night before making up our minds.'

'What made you finally decide?' I asked.

'It's difficult to say,' said Old Wang, unwilling to reveal the conflicts that had gone on in his mind. 'You see, we'd been learning about what the Chairman had to say about being unselfish and concerned about others and all that. And we knew that the couple who had bought the pig had lived just the same kind of life that we had. Another thing was that only a few days before we'd had a meeting to criticize the former brigade leader for selling a worn-out wheat grinder which had cost us 400 yuan six years ago for 300 yuan. He tried to defend himself by saying that he had not sold it on his own behalf but for the brigade as a whole and that he had not sold it to an individual but to a brigade in the next county. That was true enough, but everybody said that, whichever way you looked at it, it was just capitalist swindling and if every brigade in the country were to try and swindle every other brigade, we'd certainly never get real socialism. In the end we made him refund 150 yuan to the brigade which had bought it and since I'd voted in favour of that, how could I keep the pig just because it could find its way home?'

By chance, this was the day when the new irrigation scheme, which had involved such Herculean efforts, was due to come into operation and so, after lunch, we climbed up to the cistern cut in the rock. A small crowd of Commune members had gathered for the opening ceremony. Drums and gongs had been assembled and a choir of Young Pioneers waved their scarlet flags and sang lustily. The sun beat down from the desert of white stones on the upper slopes. The old men sat on the rocks and puffed at their long brass-bowled pipes. We waited while the workmen joined up the last section of earthenware piping. We waited while the last minutes of an epoch ticked away. We waited to see the consummation of an heroic victory.

Soon the work was finished and the oldest member of the Commune—a spruce great-grandmother of eighty-three, who still insisted on working half-day, gave the signal to start the electric motor on the other side of the hill.

Nothing happened. A tense silence gripped us. After minutes that seemed like hours, a few drops of water trickled from the pipe and disappeared into the vast empty cistern. Gradually the trickle became a torrent. Clear mountain water gushed out and echoed back faintly from the rocky depths of the cistern.

Only the children cheered.

The older ones were too moved by the magnitude of their victory over the bitter, painful past. Silently they broke up into groups and walked home.

6

Human relationships in the hospital

It is sometimes said that Communist thinking is excessively preoccupied with material things such as economics and production plans and that it pays insufficient attention to human relationships. Communism will transform human relationships and it is in order to do this that it must first revolutionize the economic structure of society. I think that China has made more progress in transforming human relationships than any country in the world and the relationships which are developing in Chinese hospitals, illustrate the direction of change.

The relationships between patients and doctors in China is based on equality and mutual respect. If both are contributing to the building of socialism, their differing contributions represent a division of labour in a common cause. There is no room for a superior or patronizing attitude on the part of the doctor and neither is there any room for the bluff heartiness, false familiarity or any other of the devices which often masquerade as a 'bedside manner'.

The doctor's job is unreservedly to serve the interests of his patients. Chinese patients, like patients all over the world, like to have things explained to them. They want to know what they are suffering from, how long it will take to get better and what treatment they are having. It is part of the doctor's duty not only to explain this fully when asked, but to volunteer such information even when not asked. This takes time, but time spent in such explanations is well spent, for reassurance and the establishment of a bond of confidence between doctor and patient play an important part in cure.

In the wards there is an informal family atmosphere very different from what I was accustomed to in England and which, at first, I found disconcerting. Now that I have got used to it, I find it natural and advantageous.

The patients often select representatives to convey their opinions and suggestions to teams of doctors, nurses and orderlies who have day-to-day responsibility in relation to specified groups of patients. These teams meet daily to plan the day's work. Ambulant patients play an active part in ward affairs. They take their meals in the ward dining-room and many of them help patients who are confined to bed, reading newspapers to them, keeping them company and becoming familiar with their medical and social problems. I conduct a ward round in a different ward each day and as I do so, I usually collect a retinue of patients who go with me, look and listen and often volunteer information. At first I thought this was an intrusion on the patient's privacy, but later I discovered that they accompanied me not out of idle curiosity but because of a genuine concern for their fellow patients and that it often helped to put me fully in the picture. Standards of privacy vary in different countries and in different social systems. Elsewhere, a woman's age and a man's income are closely guarded secrets, but in socialist China there is no reticence about such trivia.

The children in the children's ward are valuable allies in medical care. In every ward there is always at least one bright youngster who knows all about the others and who can unravel mysteries which baffle the doctors. I was perplexed by the silence of a little girl who had sustained very severe burns and who steadfastly refused to speak a word for several months. Another child explained it to me in terms that even an adult could understand. 'You see,' he said, 'when she got burned she was very frightened and thought she was going to die. Her mother and her little brother both died in that fire. Now she doesn't want to remember it and if you ask her questions and she answers them, she will remember it and feel very sad. At first she wouldn't speak to me either but now we are friends and she knows I won't ask her anything about the fire. Soon she'll start speaking to you too.' And she did.

Not only patients, but also their friends, relatives and workmates feel responsible for ensuring that everything is done in the interests of the patient. Workers who have sustained industrial injuries are brought to hospital by workmates or administrators from the factory and if the injury is serious, they often stay with them in hospital until the outcome is clear. If possible, we find beds for such escorts; otherwise they stay in a nearby inn and spend most of the day at the bedside. Mothers of young children usually live in hospital and are irreplaceable in treatment.

Medical mistakes:
A doctor's attitude to mistakes has a profound influence on the doctor/patient relationship. In China the attitude to medical mistakes is:

> prevent them
> admit them
> learn from them

Prevention is helped by the daily meetings of the groups of doctors, nurses, orderlies and patients' representatives who plan the day's work and allocate direct responsibility. All the doctors and nurses in a ward discuss major operation cases, exchanging opinions on the reasons for operation, the result to be expected, the operative procedure to be followed, difficulties that might arise during or after the operation and points to pay attention to in the post-operative period. Final responsibility rests with the surgeon in charge of the case, but the others, no matter whether they are junior or senior, are free to express their views. These discussions ensure that full preparations are made for the operation and that the post-operative care is conducted by a close knit team.

If anything goes wrong, the duty of the surgeon is to admit it frankly and never conceal it from the patient. It would be considered shameful and a betrayal of trust for a doctor to use his privileged position to deceive a patient concerning a mistake in treatment, and it would be still worse if he rallied other doctors to join him in covering things up.

The principle of learning from mistakes is deeply rooted in the work of the Chinese Communist Party. 'Taught by mistakes and setbacks, we have become wiser and handle our affairs better. It is hard for any political party or person to avoid mistakes, but we should make as few as possible. Once a

54

mistake is made, we should correct it, and the more quickly and thoroughly the better.'[1] Mishaps in treatment are, therefore, discussed both by those who were directly concerned and by others who may be involved in a similar situation in the future. Exact responsibility is traced down, not for blame but in order to learn the appropriate lessons and prevent a repetition. Very often, behind a mistake which superficially seems to be of a purely technical nature, there is a shortcoming in attitude such as a lack of responsibility, conceit, complacency or neglect of others' opinions, and the elucidation of such wrong attitudes contains lessons for everyone.

Complaints
'Even if the allegation is wrong, don't blame the allegator.'
The attitude to complaints is that, if it is justified, one should learn from it and make amends, while if it is not justified, one should not blame the patient for making it, but use it as a warning lest it become justified in the future.

Complaints by patients are, therefore, dealt with very seriously whether they are made directly to the doctor or are written in the 'Opinion Books' which are kept in every ward and department. Letters of complaint go to a special office which deals with some directly and passes others on to the person concerned. Sometimes complaints are made to newspapers, which either forward them to the hospital concerned or publish them if they have wider significance.

Litigation is very rarely resorted to, even though it is free of charge. It is unnecessary in a situation where conflicting interests between doctor and patient are reduced to a minimum, where the emphasis is on wholehearted service to patients, where every effort is made to avoid mistakes and where mistakes which do occur are freely admitted and corrected. Hospitals accept responsibility for losses incurred by patients as a result of negligence and it is not necessary to go to law about it.

Responsibility
The ideal of being 'wholly responsible' in one's attitude to patients is one which doctors of all political persuasions can readily accept. However, the criteria of what this entails differ in different social systems. For me, the concept of full responsibility has taken on a deeper meaning since coming to China. Although in the past I always thought of myself as being responsible, it is becoming clear that to be fully responsible requires more than good intentions.

I can illustrate this by referring to a patient on whom I operated recently after a mental struggle involving the principle of 'responsibility'.

He was a middle-aged peasant who had been overcome by fumes from a coal stove while cooking his supper. He had fallen unconscious across the stove and since he lived alone in a remote cottage, he remained in that position all night. His padded trousers caught fire and both legs, from the buttocks to the toes, were charred to a cinder. The little cottage was filled with hot smoke which burnt his lungs and windpipe. When he was discovered, still

[1] Mao Tse-tung, 'On the People's Democratic Dictatorship', 30 June 1949; *Selected Works, Vol. IV, p.* 422.

unconscious, the following morning, he was rushed to hospital in a critical condition. He was black in the face from asphyxia and his vocal cords were so swollen that they almost obstructed the windpipe.

Within minutes of arrival we had made an emergency opening into the windpipe to relieve the obstruction and had sucked out large quantities of frothy fluid from the lungs. With oxygen, his colour started to improve and after giving intravenous plasma, he regained consciousness.

At this point we paused to consider the problem as a whole. The outlook was extremely bad. Both lower limbs were completely destroyed from the buttocks downward and his lungs were severely burned. If he survived the next twenty-four hours he was almost certain to develop septic pneumonia and if that did not kill him, the burnt buttocks would soon become infected and, with his resistance at a low ebb, he would probably die of septicaemia. Some of the doctors thought it was impossible to save his life and doubted whether we should fruitlessly prolong his agony. If, by a miracle, he survived, he would be legless with no possibility of fitting artificial limbs since he would have no stumps.

Two fellow villagers who had brought him to hospital, as though reading our thoughts, urged us to do everything possible to save him. They explained that he was the chairman of the Association of Former Poor Peasants in his Commune, that everybody respected him for his unselfish service and would look after him very well.

We resolved to do all we could to save him and discussed our plan of treatment. It was obvious that both legs must be amputated through the hip joints, but two opposing viewpoints emerged in the course of discussion. One was that amputation should be postponed until his lungs had recovered and his general condition had improved sufficiently to enable him to withstand a very formidable operation. The other was that time was not on our side and that although early operation was dangerous, delay was even more dangerous. If we delayed, the huge burn would certainly become infected and his overall burden would be greatly increased.

Gradually, through argument, it became clear that these opposing viewpoints did not result from different estimations of the medical aspects of the case but, in essence, reflected two different attitudes towards responsibility and taking risks. No surgeon likes to run risks—especially the risk of a death on the operating table, which is distressing to the surgeon and harmful to his reputation. Of course, it is wrong to run unnecessary risks but sometimes it is safer to run a risk than to run away from it. In such cases, concern for one's reputation and peace of mind may, even though unconsciously, influence a surgeon's decisions.

We approached the problem again, determined to be guided by Mao's insistence on a full sense of responsibility and were finally able to agree that operation as soon as possible would give the best chance of survival. Accordingly, on the second day, after making very thorough preparations, we disarticulated both hips, excised the burnt skin from the buttocks and perineum and applied skin grafts to the raw areas.

The patient stood the operation remarkably well and is now able to get about in a specially modified wheel-chair. He is in good spirits and is looking forward to rejoining his fellow farmers and serving them to the best of his ability, for many years to come.

Dr Chen, an ophthalmologist from Shantung province, has related her own experiences in breaking through restrictive old orthodoxies and developing a fully responsible attitude. The orthodox treatment for serious penetrating wounds of the eyeball is removal of the damaged eye because of the danger that the remaining eye may become infected. Dr Chen, worried by the distress of patients when they were told that they would have to lose an eye, looked up medical records over many years to calculate the risk to the uninjured eye and found that infection occurred in only 0·46% of cases. Since, with modern methods of treatment it is often possible to secure a favourable outcome in cases of infection, she adopted a policy of preserving injured eyes if they retained any sense of light. As a result, partial vision has been restored in many eyes which, according to orthodox teaching, should have been removed.

She describes how, with a growing determination to be guided by proletarian politics, her attitude to blind people in her locality changed from sympathy to determination to restore vision whenever possible. So she spent hours tracking down all the blind people in the town and surrounding villages and out of a total of 219, selected fifty-three for operation. All regained some vision and one, who had been blind since childhood, strikingly illustrated the contrast between the old and the new society for, in the past, he used to beg outside that very hospital and had always been driven away with curses, whereas now, instead of being driven away, he had been sought out and invited to enter the hospital for treatment.

A veteran, who had been blinded in the revolutionary wars many years before, came to see Dr Chen with the faint hope that he might regain some degree of vision. His condition was extremely complicated and Dr Chen consulted her chief—the most experienced ophthalmic surgeon in the province. He examined the patient, looked up textbooks from all over the world and concluded that it was impossible to restore vision. But Dr Chen was not easily convinced. She remembered Mao's teaching on the relation between learning from books and learning from practice:—'Reading is learning, but applying is also learning and the more important kind of learning at that.'[1]

The realization grew that data in books can never represent anything more than the knowledge of certain men, from a certain angle, at a certain time and under certain conditions, and that most new discoveries involve unlearning what one has learned from books. She refused to be restricted within the confines of such knowledge and, after prolonged study, discussion and experimentation, she operated on the blind veteran.

This episode was subsequently presented as a stage drama and I will long remember the final scene. . . .

The time had come for removal of the bandages covering the patient's eyes. He was led into a room where the nurses and doctors who had been involved were assembled. The atmosphere was electric. As the last turn of bandage was unwound, the patient looked straight forward. He could see! And the first

[1] Mao Tse-tung, 'Problems of Strategy in China's Revolutionary War.' Dec. 1936. *Selected Works, Vol. I, pp.* 189-90.

person he saw was the elderly consultant who had declared that restoration of vision was impossible and had opposed the operation. The patient, assuming it was he who had operated on him, approached with faltering steps and grasped him by the shoulder. Choking with emotion, he said, 'The enemy blinded me. Now you have given me back my sight. I can find no words to thank you.'

The consultant, shaken out of his complacency and painfully aware that this victory had been won not by him but in spite of him, replied, 'Don't thank me. I must thank you. I too have been blind for many years but now you and Dr Chen have lifted the scales from my eyes.'

The doctor/patient relationship is, of course, a two-way relationship which also involves the attitude of the patient to his doctor and to his treatment. This, too, is changing with the changes in Chinese society and particularly under the impact of the Cultural Revolution.

I recently visited a coal-mine in Shansi province where I was told that the miners objected to having to obtain a doctor's certificate in order to go on sick leave. They said that this obsolete regulation reflected distrust of the workers. Accordingly, it was abolished and the interesting thing is that since then, the number of workers absent for health reasons has fallen sharply.

An aviator named Yuan Zhao-xiang crash-landed when his plane went out of control in a mountainous area. He sustained multiple injuries including a fracture of the spine and was not expected to resume flying. However, he was determined to do so and he co-operated so enthusiastically in all aspects of treatment that when he was told to exercise the muscles of his back, he did so with such vigour that his bed was often soaked with his sweat. To increase the effectiveness of the exercises he put weights on his shoulders and within a few weeks could raise a weight of sixty pounds in the prone position. He resumed flying duties within three months and he left a deep impression on the doctors and nurses involved in his treatment.

RELATIONSHIPS BETWEEN MEMBERS OF THE HOSPITAL STAFF

Unity

In order to weld hospital workers of all grades into a team, every member of which is dedicated to the service of patients, it is necessary to combat rivalry, selfishness and careerism, to stimulate initiative and promote thorough-going democracy. Political study, and especially study of the works of Mao Tse-tung, helps in this but to be effective, study must be linked with actual problems.

For example, some time ago a noticeably bad atmosphere developed in one of the wards in our traumatological service. Patients started complaining of indifference and carelessness and some doctors and nurses asked to be transferred to other wards.

The Party Committee asked the staff to read Chairman Mao's article 'Our Study and the Current Situation',[1] and then a meeting was held to discuss the problems in the ward in the light of this article. The meeting proceeded in a relaxed, informal manner in the ward office. An orderly started by reading

[1] Mao Tse-tung, 'Our Study and the Current Situation.' 12 April 1944. *Selected Works, Vol. III.*

aloud from the article: " 'Many things may become baggage, may become encumbrances, if we cling to them blindly and uncritically. Let us take some illustrations. Having made mistakes, you may feel that, come what may, you are saddled with them and so become dispirited; if you have not made mistakes you may feel that you are free from error and so become conceited." '

A young resident doctor, who had been sitting in a corner, interjected: 'I think that applies to me. I have made mistakes and gradually I have lost my confidence and zest for work. I missed the diagnosis in that old man with a fracture of the neck of the femur and two of my operation cases became infected. I used to be keen to be given responsibility but now I prefer safe routine jobs. I think you all look down on me and consider me a flop.'

'That's right,' said a pert young nurse. 'Many of us think you let the ward down and give it a bad name.'

'You shouldn't think that,' said the orderly who had been reading. 'Doesn't the Chairman say that the only people who don't make mistakes are those who don't do any work? It seems to me that some of you nurses have become a bit conceited because you are young and haven't made too many obvious mistakes—yet!'

The senior surgeon intervened. 'There's some truth in that,' and he went on to read from the article . . .' "Even one's age may become ground for conceit. The young, because they are bright and capable, may look down on the old; and the old, because they are rich in experience, may look down upon the young." Maybe I look down on the young from the height of my advanced age,' he said with a disarming smile.

'No, you don't do that,' said the head nurse. 'You are very nice to our young nurses and encourage them a lot. Your fault is different. The Chairman says—"Any specialized skill may be capitalized on and so lead to arrogance and contempt of others." When Dr Guo misdiagnosed the fracture of the neck of the femur, your attitude to him was very bad. Instead of explaining things to him in a comradely way, you pompously gave a lecture on the subject in front of everybody and made him feel very small. That did harm, not good.'

The discussion continued, sometimes heatedly, sometimes gently, but always with great frankness and honesty of purpose. Many simmering problems which had strained relations and impaired the work, were brought to light and analysed.

Within a few months, this ward became one of the best in hospital.

Training

Most new medical graduates take up rotating resident appointments which give them practical experience in every branch of medicine and surgery so that within a few years they are able to work independently in any field.

My own hospital has gained some reputation in traumatology and ortho-paedics and we receive a regular flow of surgeons for training in these subjects. Our post-graduate courses, both for nurses and doctors, usually last one year during which the trainees participate fully in the work and life of the hospital. They live in quarters provided by the hospital and are soon blended with our own staff who help them in every possible way.

Frequent consultations between doctors help in post-graduate training.

59

Consultations within wards on difficult cases are the rule, while more complex cases are often discussed by all doctors in the Orthopaedic and Traumatic Department at regular Saturday morning meetings. The doctor in charge of the patient reads the case history and demonstrates the physical signs after which, if the patient has no objection, those who wish to examine him, do so. Then, diagnosis and treatment are discussed, the custom being for junior doctors to speak first. In preparation for such meetings, a surgeon often analyses the results of treatment of similar patients and another may review the relevant medical literature. The hospital has a library containing medical books and periodicals from many countries and we have a special department to translate and summarize important articles. All our doctors have studied a foreign language, mostly English, and many are able to read foreign medical articles in their original language.

Consultations and 'laying eggs'

When a new hospital is built (and more than ten have been built in Peking alone since I have been here), it is staffed by transferring people from well-established hospitals on the principle (not always observed) that the best people should be transferred. The 'parent' hospital then takes on a long-term responsibility for the smooth development of the new hospital and, to help in this, senior members of its own staff may conduct regular clinics or ward rounds in the new hospital. This process of staffing and maintaining responsibility for new hospitals is called 'laying an egg'. My own hospital has laid several such eggs, some many hundreds of miles away.

In 1958, during the Great Leap Forward, the practice developed of holding nation-wide, large-scale consultations on cases presenting special problems. My own experience of such large-scale consultation was largely in the treatment of burns covering more than one half of the entire surface of the body, one of the most formidable tasks a doctor can be confronted with. China lacked experience in this field and was determined to catch up with and if possible surpass the world's most advanced levels.

I deal with this subject in more detail elsewhere. Here I will only recall the large-scale consultations which have left an indelible mark on my memory. On many occasions we assembled as many as twenty or thirty specialists in various fields to work out the best treatment for a severely burned worker. They had been invited by the Ministry of Health which arranged air-transportation for them from all over China and provided hotel accommodation for as long as necessary. Consultations often went on all night. During that time I put up a camp bed in my office so that I could snatch a few hours' sleep when the opportunity presented. I often acted as chairman at these mammoth sessions, but I lacked the tact and diplomacy necessary to give everybody a chance to air his views without prolonging the affair beyond the limits of endurance. Specialists are touchy people no matter what their nationality, and having travelled some thousands of miles, they usually feel obliged to expound their views at some length, even though what they say has already been said by others in a slightly different phraseology. It seems to be a law of nature that specialists, no matter whether they are surgeons, physicians, biochemists, endocrinologists, haematologists or bacteriologists, are firmly convinced that their field of work holds the key to success.

In retrospect, these large-scale consultations had both positive and negative aspects. On the one hand, they ensured that the most varied experience was placed at the disposal of the patient and we all learnt from each other and got to know each other. On the other hand, they were very time-consuming, they over-emphasized the importance of technique and specialized knowledge, and sometimes by the time we had agreed on a course of action, the patient's condition had changed.

Gradually the practice fell into abeyance and was replaced by another much more valuable type of collective work. This was to send out teams of doctors and nurses to supplement the local staff whenever they were asked for. They went at a moment's notice to any corner of the land. Their task was not just to consult, but to help with the actual work. When a number of steel workers in the northern steel city of Anshan sustained severe burns, a colleague and I spent more than a month there participating in the treatment and operating every day. On another occasion one of our surgeons flew to distant Sinkiang to re-operate on a patient whose severed limb had been successfully reattached but who had developed a blood clot in the joined-up artery.

Many lives and limbs have been saved and advanced knowledge and techniques widely disseminated by the nation-wide co-operation that characterizes the Chinese medical services.

DEMOCRACY versus BUREAUCRACY

Not a few foreign visitors to our hospital have commented on the democracy which is apparent even on a brief visit. I have worked in the hospital ever since it was built in 1956 and I have encountered a deep-going democracy such as I have not met elsewhere.

Doctors, nurses, orderlies, boiler-men, administrators, Party functionaries, maintenance workers and gardeners, nearly 900 of us all eat together in one huge dining-room. We collect our own food and pay for it in food tickets bought once a month. My lunch, on an average, costs the equivalent of about sixpence. We all belong to the same Trade Union, the fee for which is one per cent of the salary. No one does any private practice and everybody knows what everyone else earns.

A few years ago, the Government decided that forty-three per cent of all workers, including, of course, hospital workers, should get an increase in salary. Some guide lines were suggested as a help in deciding who should get an increase: the higher-paid should be less eligible than the lower-paid; the attitude to socialist construction should be taken into account; those with heavy family commitments and those who had not had a rise in salary for some time should get priority; working ability should be rewarded. Discussion meetings in the light of these guide lines were held in every department, and a list of names was proposed and sent to the administration. The administration made a few modifications in the light of their own estimation and sent the list back for further discussion. After several weeks of discussion, a list recommending forty-three per cent of the hospital staff for promotion was agreed and in due course they received increases in salary.

The actual level of wages and salaries in China, if translated into English currency, is low; but in my experience, very few Chinese regard themselves as being poor. In fact, they are not poor. They do not have much money but it is enough for their needs with some left over. They pay no income tax, food and clothing are cheap, rents are nominal, and frugality and plain living rather than ostentation are the order of the day.

My experience during fourteen years in China is that the Chinese people have a richer cultural life, are more articulate, use their leisure time more profitably and have a clearer understanding of where they want to go and how they are going to get there than any people I have ever met. That makes them rich, not poor.

Down with bureaucracy!

I think most of my colleagues in England would agree that doctors and hospital administrators seem to be natural enemies.

That is not so in China. All important administrative decisions are taken on the recommendation of a committee composed of elected representatives from every department. Administrative workers and Party functionaries, in accordance with regulations in force throughout China, are expected to spend one day a week doing such manual work in the hospital as sweeping the floors, stoking the furnaces or serving food. This keeps them in touch with the actual situation and is a powerful corrective for incipient bureaucracy. When a hospital director cleans a ward, he does so under the direction of the ward orderly who can form a first-hand estimate of his attitude and deflate any tendency towards superiority.

Some regard it a waste of time for a skilled administrator to clean lavatories or shovel coal. There is, in fact, a contradiction between the scarcity of trained personnel on the one hand and the requirement that they spend part of their time in relatively unskilled labour on the other.

The view of the Chinese Communist Party, however, is that the main contradiction lies not here, but in the tendency for those in positions of authority to become bureaucrats who issue orders from their offices without investigating the problems they are dealing with and who gradually put their own interests first. This tendency is very powerful and although exceptional strength of character may resist it, administrators can easily become bureaucrats unless they are confronted by a powerful corrective such as regular participation in manual labour.

The shortage of trained personnel is only temporary, but the necessity to maintain the closest links between administrators and Party functionaries and the mass of the people, and to nip bureaucracy in the bud, is permanent.

Therefore, no matter that 'Ten Thousand tasks cry out to be done. And all of them urgently', the Chinese Communist Party insists on regular participation of administrators and Party functionaries in manual labour.

My experience has been not that too much time has been spent in this way, but rather too little, since in the few years preceding the Cultural Revolution there was a tendency for this excellent practice to go by the board.

Nurses and Doctors

The relations between nurses and doctors in Chinese hospitals differ strikingly from those I encountered in England. For one thing, the sex relationship is different. Whereas in the West many young doctors regard pretty nurses as natural prey, this is not so in China. Many visitors to China regard the Chinese as being puritanical in their attitude to sex and this is understandable, for flirtatiousness is discouraged as being out of tune with the new society. This is too big a subject to be discussed here, and I will only say that there are very good historical and social reasons for the Chinese attitude to sex. Of all the tremendous changes that occurred in China after Liberation, the change in the status of women was one of the biggest. From having no rights, they became politically, economically and socially equal with men, and this transformation naturally has profoundly influenced the relationships between the sexes. A loose attitude to women is regarded not as a personal peccadillo, but as something politically reactionary. What is puritanical and what is licentious can only be decided by reference to the overall moral and political standards of society.

Many Chinese nurses are married and have children, for nursing here is not a pre-marriage interlude but an honourable lifelong career. My hospital has a day nursery for the children of all grades of hospital workers, including nurses. Naturally many nurses marry doctors working in the same hospital, but they are just as likely to marry other types of hospital workers. The relationship after marriage is also different from what it is in the West. Married women in China keep their original surnames and retain their own identity in every respect. They are never referred to as 'Mrs So-and-So,' but as 'Comrade So-and-So,' or by their full names. In the dining-room, husband and wife do not necessarily sit together but often sit with their immediate colleagues. During the Cultural Revolution, husbands and wives have sometimes found themselves in opposing political camps, in which case they attend different sets of meetings, raise different political slogans and put up sharply contrasting Big Character Posters. Usually, however, this does not affect the harmony of their private relationship.

This was illustrated during a recent ward discussion on the Cultural Revolution. Many of those present had praised a young surgeon for being politically 'left', sympathetic in his attitude to patients and professionally skilful. Towards the end of the meeting, a very pretty, kittenish young nurse who had always struck me as being shy and retiring, surprised me by speaking at length and with great passion. After sketching the course of the Cultural Revolution in the hospital, she directed her fire at the young surgeon who had been praised. 'I know he's a good doctor,' she said, 'but he's no leftist. I know what I'm talking about. He's my husband and when he comes home in the evening, he tells me all about the beautiful operations he's done, but he never tells me why he does them, whether it's to become famous or to serve the people. He reads surgical journals for hours on end, but as soon as he picks up a volume of Mao, he gets sleepy. He's quite happy to be over-burdened with clinical work so as to have an excuse for being inactive in the Cultural Revolution. He's a little hard of hearing, but whenever I speak to him about politics, he gets quite deaf. This revolution has touched most of us to the soul, but it's got nowhere near his soul. He's certainly no leftist. At best he's a middle-of-the-roader. And if he's not careful, he'll become a rightist!'

She stopped abruptly, her dimpled cheeks flushed with excitement.

It was a striking demonstration of political integrity. She loves her husband and because she loves him, she feels strongly about his political flabbiness.

There is much more equality between doctors and nurses in China than in the West. Medical students and doctors both participate in nursing work under the supervision of trained nurses. Nurses join the doctors in ward rounds and work with them in teams in which there is a division of responsibility. There is not much difference in the salary scale as between doctors and nurses and the type of accommodation provided is exactly the same.

The boundaries between their respective spheres of work are much less sharply drawn than in the West and are progressively being broken down. Chinese nurses regularly carry out procedures such as intravenous injections which are usually done by doctors in the West. More and more nurses are learning to administer anaesthetics and the operating-room nurses usually assist at operations.

Moreover, since the policy has been to orientate the health services towards the countryside, a number of experienced nurses have been selected for special training to equip them to work as doctors. This may cause some eye-brow raising among colleagues in the West and I must confess that I too experienced misgivings which no doubt reflect an habitual conservatism in medical matters.

However, after seeing the results of promoting nurses to become doctors, I am now not only reconciled to this innovation but actively support it. Common sense, devotion to the patients' interests, practical experience and a sense of responsibility are, after all, the most important requirements for medical work and there is no reason why an experienced nurse should have less of these than a young doctor just because he has studied for a few years longer. I am not belittling the importance of theoretical study. I believe that a good grasp of theory is of great value. But I agree with Chairman Mao that applying is also learning and the more important part of learning at that. Those senior nurses who are selected for training as doctors are relieved of all other duties for at least six months and go through an intensive course of medical education.

The former head nurse in our hand surgery ward has now become a doctor in the same ward. During ward rounds, I often ask her questions and she impresses me with her grasp of the complicated anatomy and physiology of the hand. She assists other surgeons in difficult operations and they assist her in simple ones. She is modest, keen to learn and dexterous, and I am sure that within a few years she will become a competent surgeon in this field.

Most nurses who become doctors are allocated work in villages, factories or mines. In the villages they are a great help to the peasant doctors who are being trained in large numbers as described elsewhere in this book. In the factories and mines they supplement the existing industrial medical service.

It is emphasized that such promotion is not a reward for talent, but a method of enabling senior nurses to increase their usefulness to the people.

In this chapter I have tried to give a picture of the relationships which exist between doctors and patients and among staff members of Chinese hospitals. What I have written is based on my own experience which is necessarily limited.

I do not want to give the impression that deeply-rooted attitudes and prejudices have been abolished as though by magic and that all problems have been solved. What has been accomplished has been the result of unremitting struggle and there is still much room for improvement. Selfishness, irresponsibility and careerism are still to be found among our medical staff. Avoidable medical mishaps still occur. Patients sometimes complain unreasonably. Some administrators and Party functionaries pay lip-service to the virtues of participation in manual labour but when it comes to the point, consistently evade it. The Trade Union, by and large, has become little more than a welfare organization.

These and other defects do not negate the essence of the situation in Chinese hospitals which is one of solid achievement and remarkable advance. All the existing defects will sooner or later be exposed and put right. Especially now, during the Cultural Revolution, everything that does not fit in with China's socialist system, everything that is shabby or second-rate, is being mercilessly criticized, discarded and supplanted.

Were I to be writing this book a few years hence, I am sure that there would still be many things to criticize, but they would not be the same things that I criticize now; I would still be able to indicate problems that cry out for solution, but they would not be the same problems that vex us now.

7

Driver Lao Li

Lao Li, our senior hospital driver, died yesterday—just after the May Day celebrations. Today, at the back of the hospital, in the open air, we held a memorial meeting for him. His photograph, draped in white, has been fixed to a decorated screen. The hospital director, a driver colleague and his second son made speeches. They told of his past—of his skill as a driver—of his devotion to duty—of his tenacity and optimism in the face of fatal illness. They spoke of his qualities as a man and as a citizen of New China.

A few days before he died he had said that when he was better, he wanted to join our mobile medical team in the mountains beyond the Great Wall, because conditions there were too rough for the second driver, who was in poor health, while the third driver was not yet sufficiently experienced for driving over dangerous mountain roads.

All around me stood hospital cooks, cleaners, nurses and doctors. Many of them were sobbing throughout the ceremony. We stood for a minute in silent mourning as Lao Li, with his untidy hair and kindly face, looked down on us from the screen festooned with gaudy wreaths of paper flowers, and then we all filed past to pay our last respects.

Lao Li had been a good friend of mine. He had driven me to and from work for many years and we always had much to say to each other. His attitude to me was that of a comrade. He had a directness that many intellectuals lack in their relationships with foreigners. To me he personified the type of ordinary Chinese worker who has benefited most from the revolution and who is completely identified with it. He sprang from a poor peasant family, had hardly any schooling, and before Liberation had come to Peking from the cold barren mountain regions where he scraped a precarious living as a carter, to try to find regular work. Eventually he became an apprentice lorry driver, sleeping beside his truck, living a life of grinding poverty and insecurity.

He went home to marry a peasant girl from his native village, returned to Peking and sent back whatever he could spare from his wages to support her and his mother. Years before, his father had been conscripted into the Kuomintang army and was never heard of again.

Whenever he was out of work he went back to his village to till the stony soil.

He had five children and never tired of telling me about them. All were at school and he was proud of them and loved them dearly. Wages are low in China and I asked him if he had any difficulty in keeping five children in school. He said he had no difficulty at all, that his expenses were trifling and he had never been so well-off in his life. In a few years' time they would graduate, and he was happy in his conviction that the education they had received would enable them to make a useful contribution to society. When I first knew him, his eldest son was studying statistics at a college in Peking. After he graduated he was appointed to a post in a woollen textile factory in Sian and once a month, when Lao Li received a letter from him, he would read it out to me.

A few years ago, while he was out with the hospital lorry collecting supplies from a town several hundred miles away, North China was hit by an unexpected deluge of rain which caused severe flooding. We were not surprised that he returned three days later than expected. He merely said that the roads were flooded and some bridges had been washed away, and we would have thought nothing more about it had we not received a letter from a People's Commune in the North China Plain asking for the name of our driver. The letter, laboriously written in a newly literate hand, described what had happened.

As Lao Li was driving through the pounding rain, the roof of a roadside granary caved in. The harvest had just been gathered and food for hundreds of families was endangered. Without hesitation he parked his truck, and undeterred by the likelihood that the entire roof might collapse, he carried sack after sack of grain to safety. When all the grain had been removed he set about ferrying homeless women and children to shelter, driving over dangerous bridges battered by swollen torrents.

For twenty-four hours he worked without rest or food and then, without saying a word to anyone, he resumed his journey back to Peking. A villager had noted the number of the lorry, traced it as belonging to our hospital and now the Commune wished to write a letter of thanks to the driver.

That's the sort of man Lao Li was, unselfish, modest, always putting the interests of others before his own. These qualities showed up in lots of little ways.

Once he bought a handsome new Chinese-made wrist-watch with a sweep second hand and a stainless steel wrist band. Before Liberation a life-time of labour could never have earned him the price of that watch—and before Liberation China had never manufactured a watch. But he needed a watch for his work, he could afford it and China was now producing watches.

A week later I noticed that he was wearing an old, shabby wrist-watch. I asked him why and he told me that he had changed watches with his daughter-in-law who was a waitress in a hotel where foreign guests often stayed. He thought it better for her to have the new watch since it would reflect credit on China's progress in light industry.

For all his steadiness, Lao Li was fully capable of losing his temper. I will long remember his anger when a driver blew a blast of his horn just as an old lady with 'lily feet' was hobbling across the road. The old lady fell down in fright and the oncoming car stopped just in time. Lao Li jumped out of his car and drenched the thoughtless driver in a torrent of invective which did full credit to his generations of cart-driver ancestors.

With the help of literacy classes in the hospital, Lao Li tried hard to keep abreast in current affairs and to master Marxism. He spent all his leisure hours studying the works of Mao Tse-tung, scanning the newspaper or reading popular novels. He would often discuss things with me, asking my opinion and disagreeing when he saw matters differently. Usually when we had a different understanding of Chairman Mao's works, he would be proved to be right and myself wrong. He used to ask me about England and showed deep feeling for the British working class.

He was unfailingly cheerful. His gratitude and devotion to the new regime was boundless and he was always telling me of the contrast with his former miserable life. He became very fond of my children and in his mind he included them with his own as part of the precious rising generation in China.

He was a true internationalist and always drew a sharp distinction between foreign friends of China and those who were hostile to China's socialist system. In 1960 he joined the Communist Party. He was often elected a model worker and then his photograph, the same as the one displayed today at the memorial meeting, would be pinned up on the notice board together with those of the other twenty or thirty model workers in the hospital.

He died of cancer of the liver complicating cirrhosis of the liver. For months his belly had been distended with fluid but he insisted that he felt well enough for light work. He said he was fed up with resting at home and wanted to do something useful. So he was given a sedentary job in the inquiry office where he soon established himself as a natural leader whose consideration for patients and their relatives was an example to all.

I saw him in the ward a few days before he died. He had wasted to a shadow and was so weak that his voice was almost inaudible. I had brought him some ice-cream and he forced a smile of thanks and said that he liked to eat cold things. We chatted for only a few minutes before his eyes closed with fatigue.

The custom of holding memorial meetings for rank-and-file comrades who die while serving the revolution started in Yenan in 1944 when Mao Tse-tung made a speech at the funeral of a charcoal burner named Chang Szu-teh. That speech, delivered in the open air to a handful of mourners, has since become famous, has been printed in millions of copies and has become a guide for the entire Chinese people. In wonderfully expressive but simple language, Mao affirmed that the greatest happiness in life lay in service to the people. All those who wholeheartedly served the people and put the people's interests before their own were great people who should be regarded as examples. When anyone who had contributed to the people's cause died, Mao said, memorial meetings should be held so that what was worthy of study could be brought out and placed before the people and so that they could express their love, their gratitude and their sorrow. In this way, the good could live on and the people become more united. In his speech, Mao quoted a Chinese historian who two thousand years before had written, 'Though Death befalls all men alike, it may be weightier than Mount Tai or lighter than a feather.' He said that the death of anyone who had truly served the people was weightier than Mount Tai.

Lao Li means Old Li but he was only forty-six when he died. We called him Old as a sign of affection. His mother, more than eighty years of age, was at his bedside when he died. She said that if she could give her life so that her son might live she would be happy. But that was not possible.

She was escorted home before the funeral because of her age and grief. She was of the old school and superstitious. She wanted an assurance that her son would not be buried in distant Peking—or worse still, cremated—but would be sent back to his native village to lie among his ancestors.

So tomorrow, Little Zheng, taught driving by Lao Li, will drive the coffin and many mourners two hundred miles through the mountains to where

Lao Li will be buried. All the funeral expenses will be borne by the hospital and Lao Li's mother will get a life pension.

Today's simple ceremony was intensely moving. I couldn't help contrasting it with my experience in hospitals in England where the death of an old hospital servant usually causes hardly a ripple. It emphasized the enormous change that had been brought about in Chinese society since I had first glimpsed it thirty years before. Then life was cheap, merely to stay alive was a triumph and the degradation of the working people knew no limit.

Today we all felt that we had lost a comrade, a man we loved and respected, a man to learn from, a man whose death was weightier than Mount Tai.

8

A marriage of East and West

When the Communists won power in 1949, they inherited a mixed medical bag. There were a number of China-trained modern-type doctors, mostly graduates of medical schools established by foreign missionaries. There were a few Chinese doctors who had trained in medical schools outside China and there were also a handful of foreign medical adventurers, doctors and self-styled doctors who, for a variety of reasons, found it safer or more profitable to live in China than at home.

No matter whether they were Chinese or foreign, most of the modern-type doctors had one thing in common; culturally and ideologically they were orientated towards the West which, in the specific conditions of old China, meant to be orientated towards Western Imperialism.

This was illustrated in an extreme form by the old Peking Union Medical College which was sponsored and controlled by the Rockefeller Foundation. On the surface, it seemed to many, including Chinese students and staff-members, to be a purely philanthropic undertaking. In fact, it trained a generation of willing henchmen who helped America to dominate China. One-quarter of the pre-1936 graduates from the Peking Union Medical College became officials in the utterly servile Kuomintang government. The health administration of that period was entirely in the hands of PUMC graduates. Responsible American officials themselves admitted that this type of penetration was cheaper and more effective than other forms.

It is, therefore, not surprising that many of the doctors trained in this kind of foreign controlled medical school shared the arrogance and acquisitiveness of their imperialist mentors. They congregated in the large cities where, as representatives of American, British, German, French or Japanese medical science, they made considerable fortunes in private practice. They set up hospitals to treat the illnesses of those who could afford to pay, and to provide refuge for warlords on the run and relaxation for harassed compradors. Although these hospitals were often staffed by Holy Sisters, they were not averse to enlisting the help of unholy sisters in providing such relaxation. Some hospitals also treated the labouring poor as charity patients, but such charity was a mixed blessing, for subsequent revelations showed that quite barbarous medical experiments were sometimes performed on unsuspecting victims.

It would be wrong to give the impression that all modern-type doctors in old China were self-seeking fortune-hunters. Many worked conscientiously and, within the limitations imposed by a corrupt and decadent society, tried to maintain a standard of medical ethics. Some, at considerable personal sacrifice, identified themselves with the common people and served them to the best of their ability. A few, including a small group of foreign doctors working in China, threw in their lot with the people's forces, worked in the liberated areas and even served in the Communist-led armies.

By far the greater part of the medical legacy consisted of traditional doctors.

Their precise number was not known for there was no binding system of medical registration, but they probably numbered about 400,000. They ranged from bearded savants of the highest culture and erudition, graduates of ancient Imperial medical schools, who could recite the medical classics by heart and write prescriptions in calligraphy of unrivalled elegance, to barely literate itinerants. Some had been apprenticed to famous doctors. Others, descended from a long lineage of healers, jealously guarded the medical lore of the clan. Still others, close to the earth of China, had grown up in the villages, spending their childhood searching for medicinal herbs on the mountain sides until, in the fullness of time, they had learned to blend, infuse and use them.

The upper crust of traditional doctors were counted among the most cultured people in old China for they were men of wide knowledge and refined tastes, connoisseurs of classical poetry, literature, painting and porcelain. They were wealthy and influential, came from big landlord families, and culturally and ideologically they were closely linked with feudalism.

The lower ranks of traditional doctors, however, were relatively close to the people. Many of them lived in county towns from which they made occasional tours through the larger villages. They charged fees which, although high for the poverty-stricken peasants, were not impossibly high and could, on occasion, be deferred or even waived.

Although most Chinese believed in traditional medicine and were deeply suspicious of the new foreign medicine with its strange jargon, the rulers of pre-revolution China, true to type, disregarded the interests of the people and in a futile attempt to drag China into what they regarded as modernity, despite the woeful shortage of modern doctors, tried to ban the practice of traditional medicine. When this failed, they obstructed it by all kinds of restrictions and forced traditional doctors out of some cities. Nonetheless, in their private lives, many of the prominent Kuomintang leaders were devotees of traditional medicine and especially of its more obscurantist and mystical aspects.

When the Communists came to power, one of the problems confronting them was to work out a policy which could unite the traditional and modern schools and utilize the services of both in the interests of the people. To understand the policy which was adopted, it is necessary to give the briefest possible outline of the content and achievements of traditional medicine.

What is traditional Chinese medicine?

The roots of Chinese medicine go back to the dawn of civilization.

The earliest and most important medical treatise was the Nei Ching, the Canon of Medicine. Tradition ascribes its authorship to Huang Ti, the legendary Yellow Emperor, believed to have lived between 2698-2598 B.C., but almost certainly it was written during the Warring States period (480-221 B.C.). The book, in eighteen volumes, is divided into two parts, the first of which is called 'Plain Questions', and the second, 'Mystical Gate'. To this day, the orthodox school of traditional medicine regards this book as its highest authority. Innumerable commentaries have been written on it and the meaning of many passages is still hotly debated.

Yin and Yang

The Nei Ching rests on two basic philosophic concepts of health and disease. The first is that normal functioning of the body depends on an equilibrium of Yin and Yang, two vital principles that permeate the whole of nature. A sunlit bank must have a bright side and a dark side; the former is Yang, the latter is Yin. One cannot exist without the other. They are mutual affinities and also mutual antipathies. In every part of the body and every biological process, Yin and Yang are operating. Yang is male, Yin is female; Yang is the back, Yin is the front; Yang the exterior, Yin the interior; the hollow organs are Yang, the solid organs are Yin. Within Yang there is something of Yin and within Yin there is something of Yang. Heat is Yang, cold is Yin. Diseases due to external causes are Yang diseases, those due to internal causes are Yin. Excessive Yang causes fever, excessive Yin causes chills. The list is endless. Every food, every medicine, every season of the year and every time of the day has a predominance either of Yin or Yang. Preponderance should not be thought of in a static, purely quantitative way, for Yin and Yang are in a constant state of ebb and flow, of imbalance seeking for balance. The question is rather which is gaining ascendancy.

The art of medicine is to ascertain where and in which direction the equipoise of Yang and Yin has been lost and then, by appropriate medication or by acupuncture, to restore it to normal.

The five elements

The second basic concept is that of the five elements and their interactions. The whole of nature, including man, consists of a mixture of five primordial substances which are exemplified in metal, wood, fire, water and earth. As long as their proportion in the body and in the various parts of the body remains normal, the body is healthy. Any disturbance in the balance results in disease, but here, too, balance must not be thought of in a static way. Some elements naturally dominate and others are dominated. Wood generates fire; fire generates earth; earth generates metal; metal generates water; water generates wood. Conversely, wood subjugates earth; earth subjugates water; water subjugates fire; fire subjugates metal and metal subjugates wood.

Traditional Chinese anatomy recognizes five solid organs each of which corresponds to one of the elements; the heart to fire, the liver to wood, the spleen to earth, the lungs to metal and the kidneys to water. Moreover, each element is related to a host of other phenomena such as the planets, colours, tastes, smells, animals, emotions, foodstuffs and climate.

The solid organs in turn are related to the hollow viscera in a particular and precise way: the lungs to the large intestine, the heart to the small intestine, the liver to the gall-bladder, the spleen to the stomach and the kidneys to the bladder.

Both solid and hollow organs respond to, and also cause, changes in the superficially placed tissues of the body: the lungs to the skin, the heart to the blood vessels of the skin, the liver to the ligaments, the spleen to the muscles and the kidneys to bone and hair.

Acupuncture

These bewilderingly complex connections and interconnections, and I have mentioned only a few of them, provide the theoretical basis for acupuncture or needle therapy, one of the three main branches of traditional medicine.

The ebb and flow of the vital Yin-Yang forces is considered to take place chiefly along twelve paired channels, six on each side, and two midline channels, one on the front and one on the back of the body. Seven of the fourteen channels are Yin and seven are Yang and along them are about six hundred named points, stimulation of any one of which will cause changes in the balance of Yin and Yang in the organ related to that point. It is interesting that there is no channel for the brain and that, as with Aristotle, the heart is thought to be the seat of consciousness.

Acupuncture consists of introducing fine metal needles into selected groups of points, often remote from the diseased organ, in order to modify the balance of Yin and Yang and give the desired result.

To help the early acupuncturists memorize the position of acupuncture points, in A.D. 1027 a life-size hollow bronze figure was cast, perforated by nearly six hundred tiny holes corresponding to them. The holes were sealed by wax and the statue filled with water so that it would be apparent when the needle had been thrust into the right place.

In the practice of acupuncture, the needles, from 4-24 cm. in length, are inserted with a twirling motion. The depth and obliquity of the needle, whether it is left still or moved while in situ, how long it remains in place—all depend on the judgment of the acupuncturist. Sometimes needling is combined with moxibustion—heating either the needle or the site of needling by holding a stick of burning moxa (wormwood or artemisia vulgaris) over it. Sometimes moxibustion is used without needling. How acupuncture works, what its indications are and how effective it is, are questions which have still to be clarified. From my own observation, I would say that it is often effective in relieving certain types of pain, sometimes quite dramatically so.

In general, practitioners of acupuncture consider that they can cure or alleviate most diseases and their great confidence may contribute in no small measure to the good results which they claim.

I well remember attending a lecture given by a peasant from Hunan who had attained a considerable reputation for his method of curing disease merely by finger pressure on the acupuncture points. He spoke with tremendous verve and enthusiasm, completely unabashed by having to confront a more or less distinguished medical audience far from his native village. He himself looked a picture of health and vitality. At the end of his talk he invited questions and I asked him whether he thought that his method could cure me of an intestinal complaint which had been defying a wide variety of modern methods. 'Of course it can,' he answered without the slightest hesitation and in full view of everybody he loosened my clothing and showed me where and how to apply finger pressure. He was certain of success and his confidence infected me. For weeks I religiously did as he had told me and, until the next attack, sure that I was cured, I enthusiastically propagandized the method among fellow sufferers. Eventually the condition cleared up, but in retrospect I find it very difficult to say whether this had anything to do with finger acupuncture.

The channels themselves are hypothetical in so far as, despite intensive research, they have not yet been demonstrated to exist as anatomical entities. Claims made elsewhere that acupuncture points can be seen microscopically, located by their electrical resistance or felt with the fingers have never been confirmed in China and are probably incorrect.

Diagnosis

Diseases are diagnosed by listening to the patient's complaints, observing his general demeanour, complexion and tongue, searching for points of tenderness along the channels and feeling the pulse. Feeling the pulse is the most important method of diagnosis and lengthy books have been written on this subject. It is maintained that the right and left pulses and the feel of the radial artery at different levels all yield different sets of information. Traditional doctors may feel the pulse for as long as half an hour before coming to a conclusion, and if the patient is in an agitated state of mind, the examination may be postponed until he has calmed down.

There are two aspects to diagnosis. One is to locate and identify the disease, to decide which organ is affected, along which channel the flow of the vital force is obstructed, where and in what way the balance of Yin and Yang has been lost. The other is to place the disease in one of four categories, namely lack or inadequacy of vital force which causes weakness and a defective reaction to the illness; excess or abnormality of vital force which causes irritability, a bounding pulse and sometimes pain; diseases of a cold nature manifested by loss of appetite, weakness of the voice and a desire for warmth; diseases of a hot nature which produce restlessness, redness of the face, dryness of the mouth and a desire for 'cold' foods, that is, foods in which the Yin principle predominates.

The category of the disease decides the basic approach to treatment; whether to stimulate or inhibit, to supplement or to dissipate, to warm or to cool, to boost the Yin or the Yang. The location of the disease determines the technique; whether to use needling or moxibustion alone or in combination, which acupuncture points to use, what drugs to give, what diet to prescribe.

Traditional Chinese drugs

The theoretical basis of Chinese medicine was, in essence, worked out some two thousand years ago, and since then the chief development has been the discovery of new drugs to alter the balance of Yin and Yang. A veritable multitude of herbs, minerals and animal products has been tested out during the intervening centuries.

The Shen Nung Materia Medica, written about the first century B.C., listed more than three hundred remedies including mercury and sulphur for skin diseases. Three hundred years later, in 'Medical Principles and Essentials', some eighty additional medicaments including antipyretics, cathartics, diuretics, emetics, sedatives, stimulants, digestive remedies and anti-diarrhoeal drugs were described.

In 1578, after twenty-seven years of research, the great pharmacologist Li Shih-chen published his 'Compendium of Materia Medica', a scientific masterpiece which listed 1,892 drugs and some ten thousand prescriptions.

One thousand and ninety-four of the drugs were of vegetable origin, four hundred and forty-four zoological and the remainder mineral. He classified them into sixteen classes and sixty-two divisions according to their biological characteristics and pharmaceutical value thus making a notable contribution both to pharmacology and biology. Many of the drugs he used, such as Iodine, Kaolin, Ephedrine for asthma, Dichroa febrifuga for malaria and Mylitta lapidescens for tape-worm, are still in use today.

The achievements of traditional medicine

Seen in the light of modern scientific discoveries, the theories of Chinese traditional medicine seem irrational and dogmatic. However, at the time they were put forward they embodied brilliant deductive reasoning based on empirical observation.

Looking back over the centuries, traditional medicine has much to its credit.

The Canon of Medicine, around two thousand years before Harvey's monumental proof of the circulation of the blood, stated: 'The blood current flows continuously in a circle and never stops. It may be compared to a circle without beginning or end.'

The same book placed great stress on preventive medicine, affirming that curing a disease is 'like digging a well after one has become thirsty', or like 'forging weapons after the battle has begun'. It advocated prevention of disease by regular habits, proper diet, a suitable combination of work and leisure and the maintenance of a calm mind. This may sound elementary, but it should be remembered that a thousand years later the concept of disease prevention had hardly reached the Western world where illness was still widely regarded as a punishment for sin.

Surgery attained a high level during the Han dynasty. Hua To, the ablest surgeon of his day, performed major operations under general anaesthesia and worked out an excellent system of remedial exercises based on imitating the movements of the tiger, the stag, the bear, the monkey and the bird. According to the Romance of the Three Kingdoms, he met his doom when he was consulted by Ts'ao Ts'ao, the despotic prime minister who was complaining of severe headache. Hua To diagnosed a tumour of the brain and proposed an operation, but the suspicious Ts'ao Ts'ao sensed a plot to assassinate him and had Hua To executed. However, the description of Ts'ao Ts'ao's own demise suggests that Hua To's diagnosis was probably correct.

The Imperial Institute of Physicians, set up by Tang dynasty emperors in the seventh century A.D., was the first medical school in the world. It had an enrolment of some 350 students specializing either in medicine, acupuncture or surgery—the three divisions of traditional medicine. Surgery included skin diseases, haemorrhoids, and the treatment of fractures, wounds and septic conditions.

China's first hospital was established in A.D. 510 to cope with an epidemic in Shansi province, and during the following centuries a number of Government-organized hospitals for lepers and the sick-poor were set up.

Smallpox, then a devastating epidemic disease, attracted great attention and more than fifty ancient treatises were written on this subject. In the middle of the sixteenth century, over 200 years before Jenner's epoch-making discovery, a form of inoculation against smallpox consisting of extracting and drying the contents of a pustule from a smallpox victim and blowing the powder into the nose, gained wide acceptance in China. Russian doctors came to China to study this method in the seventeenth century and news of it reached England in 1717.

Despite its rudimentary anatomy and physiology, traditional medicine clearly had great achievements to its credit and was still capable of making a valuable contribution to preserving the health of the Chinese people. It had accumulated a vast store of accurate observations and empirical knowledge which, notwithstanding its overlay of dogma and superstition, contained much that was of value. What was needed was to sift the gold from the dross and put a refined and rejuvenated system of traditional medicine at the service of the people.

A new policy

At the heart of the medical problem was the fact that China had too few modern-type doctors and that most of the few were more concerned with making money than with looking after the disease-ridden, poverty-stricken peasant masses.

On the other hand, there were some hundreds of thousands of traditional doctors. The people believed in traditional medicine and although its theory had not yet completely broken free from the shackles of the past, it still had a contribution to make and, given the right kind of stimulus, was capable of big advances.

As early as 1944, while the anti-Japanese war was still in progress, Chairman Mao had worked out a correct policy in relation to traditional medicine. He wrote: 'Among the 1,500,000 people of the Shensi-Kansu-Ningsia Border Region, there are more than 1,000,000 illiterates, there are 2,000 practitioners of witchcraft, and the broad masses are still under the influence of superstition . . . the human and animal mortality rates are both very high. . . . In such circumstances, to rely solely on modern doctors is no solution. Of course, modern doctors have advantages over doctors of the old type, but if they do not concern themselves with the sufferings of the people, do not unite with the thousand and more doctors and veterinarians of the old type in the Border Region and do not help them to make progress, then they will actually be helping the witch doctors. . . . There are two principles for the united front: the first is to unite, and the second is to criticize, educate and transform.'[1]

Within a year of Liberation, he succinctly expressed the same policy in a directive to the First National Health Conference: 'Unite all medical workers, young and old, of the traditional and Western schools, and organize a solid united front to strive for the development of the people's health work.'

To a greater or lesser degree, despite the resistance of those who paid lip-service to the policy while opposing it in practice, it has been implemented politically, organizationally, educationally and scientifically.

[1] 'The United Front in Cultural Work.' *Selected Works, Vol. III. Peking.*

Politically, it expressed itself in a campaign to unite all medical workers in a common desire to serve the people and contribute to China's socialist construction. Political study helped them to understand the source of the antagonisms which existed between the traditional and modern schools and to arrive at a correct attitude to traditional medicine as a part of their country's cultural heritage. It helped them to steer clear of the twin pitfalls of a narrow nationalism which uncritically praised everything indigenous, and a slavish acceptance of anything foreign just because it was foreign.

Organizationally it expressed itself in concern for the rights and status of traditional doctors. They now have the same rights, the same protection and the same rewards as modern doctors of equal standing. In the early years they mostly worked in individual private practice, but group practice gradually supplanted individual practice and in recent years many of the group practices have come under state control. Many traditional doctors have been enrolled on the staffs of modern hospitals, working side by side with their modern-type colleagues, co-operating with them in every way. My own hospital has a full complement of traditional physicians, acupuncturists and manipulative surgeons, whom we often consult in the treatment of patients. Traditional doctors have access to modern diagnostic methods such as X-rays and laboratory investigations and modern-type doctors help them to use these facilities. Hospitals exclusively for the practice of Chinese medicine have been built, incorporating features new to traditional medicine, such as case-history filing departments.

Educationally the policy expressed itself by including courses on traditional medicine in the curriculum for medical students of the modern school and by ensuring that their internship includes practical work under experienced traditional doctors. Large numbers of young modern-type doctors have attended short courses in traditional medicine and some senior physicians have been given the opportunity for intensive study for periods of one or two years. Although traditional doctors were urged to learn something of modern medicine, the main emphasis has been on modern doctors learning traditional medicine and not vice versa. Simplified books on traditional medicine have been published and most out-patient departments display charts showing acupuncture points. The training of traditional doctors is becoming standardized and many new traditional medical schools have been built.

Scientifically the policy expressed itself in research work along two main lines. One was to analyse and test the efficacy of traditional remedies and try to find out how traditional methods, including acupuncture, work. This type of work is largely done in research institutes by teams of traditional and modern doctors, pharmacologists, biochemists, physiologists and laboratory workers.

The other is to conduct clinical research into methods of blending traditional and modern medicine with the object of evolving a new type of medicine, superior to either alone. This is mostly done in general hospitals by modern-type doctors working in co-operation with traditional practitioners. It is a kind of research which, because it concerns itself more with practice than with theory, is able to achieve relatively quick results which, in turn, can open up fruitful avenues for basic theoretical research.

77

Integrated fracture treatment

The integration of traditional and modern methods in the treatment of fractures is a field in which I have had some personal experience. I shall therefore use it to illustrate this type of research.

The first Chinese book on the treatment of fractures, which appeared in the ninth century A.D., laid down principles of treatment which are still observed by traditional surgeons and which stand in sharp contrast to those which have come to be widely accepted in Western countries.

Since traditional methods of treating fractures have been in use for more than a thousand years, there can be no doubt that they must in general have been successful or they would long since have been discarded. A patient may not know if his gastric ulcer has healed, but he certainly knows whether his fracture has united. Our task was to compare the validity of traditional and modern principles of fracture treatment, to find the strong and the weak points of each and to combine them in such a way that the result would be better than either alone.

There are three main differences between the two approaches to the treatment of fractures.

The modern school usually aims to reduce the fracture—to bring the two ends of the broken bone into normal alignment—in a single manipulation, usually forcible and therefore carried out under anaesthesia. The traditional school aims to achieve this gradually, step by step, without the use of anaesthesia.

The modern school usually immobilizes the broken bone as completely as possible until it has firmly united. The traditional school does not regard immobilization as essential or even as particularly desirable and it uses splints not to prevent movement, but to prevent a recurrence of displacement after the fracture has been reduced.

The modern school, in order to achieve maximum immobilization, usually also immobilizes the joints above and below the fracture. For example, if the fracture is in the leg, the knee and ankle joints are usually immobilized until the fracture has united. The traditional school, on the contrary, insists on the freedom of joints above and below the fracture, maintaining that their immobilization is both unnecessary and harmful, causing joint stiffness and muscle wasting and slowing down or even preventing healing of the fracture.

It would be wrong not to point out, at this stage, that the 'modern school' is by no means a monolithic bloc within which everybody agrees. There are clashes of opinion, sometimes very sharp ones. Moreover, since different fractures require different treatment, there can be no such thing as a standard treatment for all fractures.

Notwithstanding this, the principles of quick reduction and complete, uninterrupted immobilization by plaster of Paris casts which immobilize the joints above and below the injury, are undoubtedly the dominant principles guiding the treatment of fractures in the West.

The traditional method of treating fractures essentially consists of coaxing the broken ends into alignment by gentle finger pressure and then tying short splints of malleable wood around the limb sufficiently tightly to maintain the alignment. The pressure of the splints is concentrated where most desired by placing springy pads of folded paper beneath the splints, the pads being held in place by a layer of sticky medicinal paste which is also thought to help the swelling to subside. Usually the splints are removed the next day and the position of the broken ends is determined by observing and feeling the limb. If reduction is not complete, the position is improved by finger pressure and the splints are reapplied. When reduction is satisfactory, daily inspection is discontinued, but the tightness of the tapes which encircle the limbs needs constant readjustment as the swelling subsides.

Exercises of the injured limb are started as soon as reduction is satisfactory and are usually combined with traditional Chinese callisthenics to the whole body. All joints are left free and the patient is encouraged to move them actively. Traditional doctors usually give their fracture patient pills containing herbal remedies and certain mineral substances which are thought to expedite healing of the bone, but it is doubtful whether they actually do so.

It soon became clear to us that purely traditional methods of fracture treatment had good and bad aspects.

The main advantage was that most fractures united more quickly and more certainly than if they had been treated with plaster of Paris casts. The method was free from all the risks of open operation and it used materials which were cheap and universally available. Anaesthesia was unnecessary and muscle wasting and joint stiffness were minimized. Most simple uncomplicated fractures treated by traditional methods recovered normal function very quickly.

On the other hand, there were drawbacks. It was not always possible to reduce the fracture by simple finger pressure without anaesthesia and neither was it always possible to prevent redisplacement after reduction. Oblique and fragmented fractures were difficult to control and sometimes united with excessive shortening. The method was troublesome and time-consuming and many fracture cases which would have been treated as out-patients in the West, required hospitalization for close observation, repeated reduction and readjustment of the splints. If the splints were tied too tightly, sloughing of the soft tissues and other serious complications could result, and although mishaps of this kind also occur with modern methods and are not inherent in the method itself but are due to its misuse, they occurred frequently enough to cause some misgivings.

We carried out many animal experiments which tended to confirm that fractures united more quickly with local splint fixation than with long plaster casts. A method of estimating the richness of the blood supply in and around the broken bone ends by filling the blood-vessels with radio-opaque material, showed that new blood vessels sprouted more abundantly in fractures treated by traditional methods, that callus formed earlier and in larger amounts, and that the haematoma between the broken bone ends was changed into living tissue more quickly.

Gradually we evolved new methods of treatment combining the advantages of each school. Fractures with a tendency to shortening were treated by a period of traction as is used in the modern school, but this was combined with traditional splintage to control the position of the fragments, and early movements of the injured limb were encouraged. The duration of traction was much shorter than it would have been with modern methods alone, and weight-bearing, in fractures of the lower limb, was permitted at an earlier phase of union.

The straight wooden splints which had been used for centuries, were changed for moulded splints, thus spreading the pressure and reducing the risk of pressure sores. Some hospitals used short splints made of plaster of Paris, moulded to fit the individual patient with the same objective.

The actual pressure necessary to maintain the position of the broken ends at different stages was measured experimentally and methods were devised for ensuring that this pressure was not exceeded.

In the treatment of some fractures, it was found that aspects of both methods could be combined throughout treatment while, in others, it was better to start with modern methods and change to traditional methods after a few weeks. Some fractures were best treated by traditional methods alone, while others, particularly compound fractures in which one of the bone ends had protruded through the skin, were best treated by modern methods.

Gradually we are coming to understand how to combine the strong points of each method so as to improve our overall results and although no nation-wide method of integration has yet been worked out and different hospitals use different methods, most surgeons in China now use integrated methods to treat fractures. A hospital in Tientsin has reported that by using a combination of modern and traditional methods, it has halved the time necessary for healing of fractures of the upper arm and ankle and reduced the time for healing of leg fractures to slightly less than half.

In my opinion, some caution is needed in accepting these claims in their entirety for there are so many variables, so many factors to be taken into account, including the surgeon's subjective estimation of when a fracture can be said to have united, that reliable comparisons are difficult to make and may be wrong. What can be safely said is that simple fractures treated by integrated modern and traditional methods unite more quickly and with more certainty than with modern methods alone. Work is still continuing along these lines and will continue for many years to come. I feel convinced that what will finally emerge will constitute an advance in the treatment of fractures.

The policy of promoting unity between the traditional and modern schools and of combining the best of both, is a correct policy which is benefiting the Chinese people and which, in the fullness of time, will enrich medical science. Traditional Chinese medicine is the oldest medical system in the world. At a time when most countries were still uncivilized, it had reached a high level, and during the centuries it accumulated a wealth of new observations and discoveries which were recorded in minute detail.

Then, at a certain stage, encrusted with superstition and dogma, it became dormant. Modern medicine arose in the West and its scientific achievements soon surpassed those of traditional medicine.

Today, New China, in its political essence the most modern society in the world, has awakened traditional medicine from its long sleep and brought about a marriage between the old and the new. The new is rejuvenating the old and the old is enriching the new. It is devoutly to be hoped that this marriage will generate a new and vigorous system of medicine, better than either of its forebears, capable of serving the needs of all mankind.

9

The conquest of syphilis

On a blustery day in December, 1920, a strange farce was enacted in the Town Hall in the International Settlement of Shanghai.

There had been some difference of opinion as to whether or not children should be admitted to the ceremony. Some had been against it lest it sully their pure little minds with unwholesome thoughts and cause them to ask awkward questions. But the majority had been in favour. 'After all,' they argued, 'there is little enough entertainment for children in this wicked city and Christmas is but four days ahead. The dear little innocents won't understand what is going on and it will give them a chance to plan their Christmas parties.'

There were no two opinions as to whether or not Chinese should be admitted. 'Let us fling our civic doors wide open,' declared the vicar magnanimously. 'Let us welcome spectators of all colours, creeds and denominations. Let us show them every courtesy and every hospitality. Some of them, inspired by the proceedings, will draw closer to us. Moreover, they will all pay the entrance fee and so assist our all-too-modest welfare fund.'

The wife of a High Court judge who had consented to draw the lots, took her seat beside the lottery drum. Her poise and grace contrasted with the evident embarrassment of the few brothel-keepers sitting at the back of the platform. No more than twenty had come out of the nine hundred who had been invited and they had not expected to be let down in this way by their professional colleagues. Neither had they expected to have those ridiculously huge paper roses pinned on to their lapels or to be showered with prayer books, religious tracts and crucifixes. Above all, they had not expected that the ceremony would take so long, for the festive season was approaching and they were busy men.

Her ladyship drew slips of paper from the drum and the moderator read out the names inscribed on them. At first, each name was greeted by a ripple of applause but soon the audience lost interest and a hum of conversation filled the chilly hall. When 180 names had been read out, a Civic Dignitary made a little speech in which he thanked all those who had participated and especially the 180 brothel keepers who were now in honour bound to close their establishments and free 1,200 girls by next April. He had prepared a much longer speech calling attention to the epoch-making nature of the proceedings and to the implications which they held for the moral and physical welfare of the Settlement, but he sensed that a long speech at this late hour would not meet with universal approval.

Only one of the brothel keepers actually present had had his name called out and he took it remarkably well. He grinned sheepishly as his colleagues either sympathetically patted him on the back or hypocritically shook his hand in congratulations. He mopped his brow from time to time in spite of the cold, fidgeted with his rosette and the only thing at all unseemly in his behaviour was when he peeped into the drum to see whether it could possibly have contained all nine hundred names.

Not that he was worried. He knew perfectly well that most of the names that had been called out were fictitious. But he, having a reputation to keep up, wouldn't stoop to such a low trick. His establishment anyway needed redecorating and he would need only to change the signboard and install his brother as the proprietor. What queer notions some people had! To expect a brothel keeper voluntarily to close down a flourishing concern was like expecting the police to entrust the keys of the jail to the inmates.

But it was as well to play ball with civic big shots, time-consuming though it was. You never could tell when you would need their help.

The National Medical Journal of China at first hailed the event as a 'red-letter day for social reformers in Shanghai',[1] but later it editorialized: 'As we said in our last issue, we hope the French municipal authorities will come into line. With the present tendencies in world thought, civic authorities cannot afford to ignore the moral and physical welfare of millions of people *entrusted* to their care, *even though* they be of another race and nationality' (author's italics). The background to this sanctimonious gem was the fact that the French 'Concession', which accommodated slightly more than half of all the registered brothels in Shanghai, had not participated in this particular tragi-comedy.

Not that it would have made much difference if they had, since a conservative estimate of the number of prostitutes in Shanghai at that time was 50,000 registered and 100,000 unregistered.

The history of venereal disease in China

Until 1504, venereal disease was unknown in China, and this was not because it had not yet been correctly diagnosed, for at that time Chinese Traditional Medicine was already well advanced and hundreds of diseases had been accurately described in manuscripts which are still extant.

In that year, the old colonialists introduced syphilis into Canton and it soon spread widely throughout the whole land.

Syphilis is a 'social disease'—that is, a disease whose incidence and spread (and, as we shall see, its decline and eradication) are dependent on social and political factors. What were the political and social factors responsible for the hold it gained in China?

Firstly, imperialism and colonialism, the forcible occupation of her territory by invading countries, the subjugation of her people and the wrecking of her economy. In 1877, more than three hundred years after the introduction of syphilis into Canton, the British Admiral in Shanghai, concerned about the mounting incidence of venereal disease among the sailors under his command, summoned his Surgeon-Commander and between them they devised a scheme to protect them. They instituted a totally illegal system of compulsory medical examination of prostitutes with a fee for examination and a money fine for non-compliance. In the first year the revenue from fines and fees totalled 2,590 taels of silver. But the syphilis rate was unchanged.

Secondly, war, inseparable from imperialism and from the fragmentation of Chinese society consequent upon it.

[1] *Nat. Med. Journ. of China, No.* 6, 1920, *p.* 226.

Invading armies, and indigenous armies in the service of exploiters and oppressors, habitually loot, ravage and rape. They become infected with syphilis and they spread syphilis. The Kuomintang armies had a syphilis rate of about twenty per cent.[1] The incidence of syphilis in Chinese villages was directly proportional to the size and the duration of stay of invading US, Japanese and Kuomintang armies.

Thirdly, poverty, a result of feudal and capitalist exploitation and of the economic backwardness and insecurity they caused.

The editorial of the National Medical Journal of China for September 1920, entitled 'Vice, Famine and Poverty,' reads as follows:

'. . . The year 1920, will, we fear, be marked by much suffering, especially in the North where the long drought killed most of the crops and thus brought 20 *million* people to the verge of starvation. The present famine will swell the ranks of slave girls and prostitutes.'[2]

Fourthly, drug addiction. Until the British East India Company sent the first big shipment of Indian-grown opium into China in 1781, the drug was almost unknown in China. For many years before then, British merchants had bought Chinese tea, silk, cotton-textiles, porcelain and manufactured goods of a quality and variety unknown elsewhere, but in return, China imported very little. Replying to a proposal for wider trade, the Emperor Chien Lung wrote to King George III of England: 'We possess all things. I set no value on things strange or ingenious and have no use for your country's manufactures.' So the British merchants had to pay for China's exports in the silver which they had obtained by selling slaves in silver-rich Mexico and Peru. To halt this drain on their silver, the British East India Company extended the cultivation of the opium poppy in Northern and Central India and boosted sales to China. By 1820, profits from the sale of opium accounted for twenty per cent of the revenue of the British government of India. China's annual imports of opium rose from 2,000 chests (140-160 pounds in each) in 1800 to 40,000 chests in 1838, and silver flowed out of China at such a rate that, between 1832 and 1835, twenty million ounces left the country.

In self-preservation, the Chinese rulers had to act. On 3 June, 1839, Lin Tse-hsu, the special commissioner for Canton, forced the British and American opium merchants to hand over 20,000 chests of opium which he publicly burned. The result was the First Opium War ending in the humiliating Treaty of Nanking (1842) which ceded Hong Kong, opened the door wide to imperialist penetration and guaranteed a huge and exceedingly profitable market for the sale of narcotics.

'Legal' importation of opium into China continued until 1917 and after that 'illegal' importation continued until Liberation in only slightly reduced amounts and at a very much higher rate of profit.

Dr L. T. Wu, engaged in Narcotic Control in 1920, complained: 'What can Chinese government regulations do when advanced countries like Britain and the USA produce and export unlimited quantities of morphine and

[1] Lai, D. G., et al. 'Incidence of syphilis among Chinese Soldiers in Swatow.' *Chinese Med. Journal*, 42, 557, 1928.

[2] *Nat. Med. Journ. of China, Sept.* 1920. *Vol. VI, No.* 3.

heroin without any question or supervision of their destination and when there are post-offices throughout China over which the Chinese Government has no control? . . .'[1]

Drugs and prostitution are co-partners in depravity. Most brothels were also opium dens and the girls, who had been sold into prostitution at an early age and who were not free to leave, also became addicts and lost their will to resist.

Fifthly, an attitude to women characteristic of class society which sees women as inferior to men, as their chattels and playthings. In feudal society with its polygamy, concubinage, child-marriage and a complete absence of legal and property rights for women, there was no attempt to disguise the inequality between the sexes. In Western capitalist society, where the legal trappings of equality exist to a greater or lesser degree, the inferior status of women still persists in a concealed form, and organs for moulding public opinion, from glossy magazines to television, inculcate an obsessive pre-occupation with sex and present a picture of woman as little more than the sum total of her vital statistics.

World-wide trends in venereal disease

We have seen that the spread of venereal disease in China was closely connected with policies pursued by 'advanced' imperialist countries.

What was happening within these countries themselves? In 1905, Paul Ehrlich, after 606 experiments, discovered the world's first chemotherapeutic drug, Salvarsan, which he named 606. It was thought that one dose would cure syphilis and it was hailed as a beneficent contribution to civilization. Some, however, were less enthusiastic. If veneral disease can be so easily cured, they argued, then this drug will become a license for lechery; venereal disease will disappear but fornication will flourish. They need not have worried. Venereal disease did not disappear. Neither did it after Penicillin, a much more potent drug, was discovered. It takes more than drugs to eliminate syphilis just like, as the Vietnamese are showing, it takes more than weapons to win a war.

Since 1957, syphilis has continually increased in the USA where there are at least 1.2 million *untreated* cases.[2]

According to minimal official estimates, the venereal disease rate among the invading US forces in Vietnam in 1966 was ten per cent[3] although other estimates put the figure as high as forty per cent. The incidence is still increasing, for in the first six months of 1967, 46,561 *new* cases of venereal disease were reported among US troops in Vietnam as compared with 27,701 cases for the same period the previous year.[4] Venereal disease ranks highest of six major diseases among US troops in Vietnam.

[1] *Nat. Med. Journ. of China No.* 6, 1920, *p.* 66.

[2] Clark, E. G. 'Untreated Syphilis and Natural Course.' *Proceedings 12th International Congress of Dermatology*, 2. 855. *Washington.*

[3] *US News and World Report. May* 1966.

[4] *US News and World Report.* 16 *October,* 1967. *p.* 37.

There has been a huge increase in venereal disease in Australia in the past six years.

A Christchurch specialist, Dr W. M. Platts, states that 'last year sixty per cent of New Zealand girls attending VD clinics were under the age of twenty —a proportion approached only by Sweden. . . . In 1955 the disease seemed to be under medical control . . . but since then the incidence of gonorrhoea has passed the peak reached in the 1930s. It had risen not only in New Zealand but in most parts of the world.'

VD in Britain, especially among teenagers, has been rising alarmingly and is now the second largest group of notifiable diseases after measles. The incidence of gonorrhoea doubled in a decade and that of infectious syphilis trebled in the six years up to 1965. Venereologist Dr Catterall of the Middlesex Hospital, London, describes the world-wide epidemic of venereal disease as 'one of the major health problems of the second half of the twentieth century'.

In 1963, Ambrose King and Claude Nichol, president and vice-president respectively of the International Union against VD, stated:[1] 'Shortly after the Second World War there were high hopes that the venereal diseases were nearing extinction, and it has been a surprise to many that in a settled and prosperous society at peace and with potent therapeutic agents to hand, these diseases should be causing anxiety. In recent years there has been an increase in the incidence of syphilis and gonorrhoea in many countries. . . . At any rate, it seems that the problem of the venereal diseases is with us for the foreseeable future.'

The incidence of VD in pre-Liberation China

Since the Kuomintang health authorities left behind no reliable official statistics, estimates of its pre-Liberation incidence must be based either on figures published at the time by individual research workers or on conditions which were found to exist soon after Liberation.

In most National Minority areas[2] the incidence of syphilis was more than ten per cent. There were many reasons for this very high incidence including poverty, ignorance, superstition and oppression by their own feudal rulers, by Han landlords and merchants and by marauding war-lords. Many of these National Minority societies were very primitive and, in some, slavery was only abolished after Liberation. Feudal lords and religious leaders (the latter nominally celibate) took what women they wished and spread venereal disease far and wide. There were no medical services to speak of and what there were, were beyond the reach of ordinary persons.

The offspring of the feudal or religious aristocracy were habitually put out to be wet-nursed by slave or serf women and, if the babies had congenital syphilis, they infected their wet-nurses.

[1] King, A., and Nichol, C. *Venereal Diseases, ed. I, pp.* 7-9, *Cassel, London*, 1964.

[2] These are regions of the People's Republic of China where the majority of the inhabitants are of non-Han nationality. They have their own language, dress, religion and customs. Although they number no more than 6% of the Chinese people, the territories in which they have regional autonomy cover some 60% of the area of the Chinese People's Republic and 14·6% of deputies to the National People's Congress are members of National Minorities.

In cities and urban areas, the incidence was five per cent and in the countryside it averaged between one and three per cent. However, in those rural areas ravaged by the Kuomintang armies, it was much higher.

When one recalls that China has a population of seven hundred million, the magnitude of the problem becomes clearer. There were some tens of millions of syphilitics scattered throughout the country, most of them suffering from latent syphilis but many still potentially infectious.

The present venereal disease situation in China

The present position can be stated in one short sentence.

ACTIVE VENEREAL DISEASE HAS BEEN COMPLETELY ERADICATED FROM MOST AREAS AND COMPLETELY CONTROLLED THROUGHOUT CHINA.

This is a sweeping statement but I am convinced that it is true.

I now give some fragments of the vast mass of facts on which it is based.

In Peking it is impossible to find active syphilitic lessons to demonstrate to medical students. A generation of doctors is growing up in China with no direct experience of syphilis but this is of little consequence for the disease will never return.

At a conference held in the Research Institute of Dermatology and Venereal Disease of the Chinese Academy of Medical Sciences in January 1956,[1] specialists from eight major cities reported that a total of only twenty-eight cases of infectious syphilis had been discovered in their areas in the four years 1952-55. An investigation of infectious syphilis in seven major cities between 1960 and 1964 showed that by the end of this period, the early syphilis rate was less than twenty cases per hundred million of population per year; that is, it had very nearly reached the point of extinction.

In the National Minority areas, especially in those where the syphilis rate had been highest, a striking fall occurred in the ten years between 1951 and 1960. In the Wulatechien Banner of Inner Mongolia, where the syphilis rate had been nearly fifty per cent in 1952, not a single case of infectious syphilis was found among 3,158 persons examined at random in 1962. In the Jerimu Banner of the Djarod League, which had shown a sero-positivity rate of thirty-five per cent in 1952, ninety-seven per cent of the whole population was tested for syphilis and not a single new, infectious or congenital case was found.

Before Liberation, one of the harmful effects of the widespread syphilis in Minority areas was a progressive depopulation resulting from lowered fertility, a high miscarriage rate and the large number of babies born dead.

For example, the Ikechao League in Inner Mongolia, which had a population of 400,000 in the seventeenth century, was reduced to 80,000 persons by the time of Liberation. The Hulunbu League, which numbered 10,386 in 1933, had fallen to 7,670 in 1950 and an investigation of 2,334 nomadic families revealed that fifty-eight per cent were childless.

Following the anti-syphilis campaign this depopulation trend was reversed

[1] Dr Ma Hai-teh, *China's Medicine. No. 1. Oct. 1966.*

In the Djarod Banner the population increased from 2,548 to 3,343 in ten years. In the same period, 390 herdsmen's families in Hulunbu League, Wusumu, registered increases of from 14·1 per cent to 21·6 per cent.

My friend Dr Ma Hai-teh, who has actively participated in the anti-syphilis campaign since its inception and to whom I am indebted for much of the material in this chapter, tells me of a Mongolian woman suffering from syphilis who had been married for five years but had not given birth to a live child. She was given a course of treatment in 1952 and the following year she demanded more injections because after the first course she had given birth to a fine baby boy and she wanted another. Tests showed that she had been cured and she was not seen again until the ten-year follow-up when she appeared with eight children, having left one at home. This time she stated flatly that whatever the doctors said, she would have no more injections. She now had a big enough family and was satisfied!

In the rural areas, intensive search shows that the disease has been virtually eliminated. In Hsingku and Ningtu counties in Kiangsi province, a follow-up study five years after the anti-syphilis campaign revealed no new cases or recurrences. In 1960, a complete dermatological examination of the entire population in Chaoan county (population 746,495) Kwangtung province, and Haian county (population 225,305) Kiangsu province, revealed only one case of secondary recurrent syphilis, and a re-survey of fifty per cent of the population of these two counties in 1964 showed not a single infectious case.

How the victory was won

Since, as has been shown, the spread and persistence of syphilis in any country is due to social and political factors, it can only be eliminated by tackling these factors. That is to say, only an all-round political, as opposed to a purely technical, medical or legislative approach, can ever solve the problem.

The conquest of syphilis in China within a few years of the conquest of power by the Chinese working class is an outstanding example of the decisive role of politics in tackling major health problems.

There were two essential preconditions for the elimination of syphilis from China. The first was the establishment of the socialist system which ended exploitation and made the oppressed masses the masters of their fate. The second was the equipping of all those involved in the campaign, whether lay or medical, with a determination to serve the people and help socialist construction, with the method of thinking of Mao Tse-tung, so that they would be able to surmount all difficulties confronting them.

The following measures were carried out on the basis of these two prerequisites:

The elimination of prostitution

Within a few weeks of Liberation, most of the brothels were closed down by the direct action of the masses. The vast majority of the people recognized that prostitution was harmful and that it constituted crude exploitation of the prostitutes who, for the most part, had been driven into prostitution by poverty or by brute force. Brothel keepers who were scoundrels, drug-peddlers or gangsters were dealt with directly by the angry masses or handed over to the Public Security forces. The few remaining brothels were closed down by Government order in 1951 when prostitution was made illegal.

The prostitutes were treated as victims of an evil social system. First it was necessary to cure the venereal diseases which affected more than ninety per cent of them and then to embark on their social rehabilitation. Those who had been prostitutes for only a short time were encouraged to go home and were found jobs. It was patiently explained to their families that no shame was attached to having been a victim of the old society and that now everyone who did an honest job was worthy of respect. Those who were deep rooted in prostitution were asked to enter Rehabilitation Centres where they studied the policy of the Government towards them, the nature of the new order, the reasons why they had become prostitutes and the new prospects which were opening up for them providing they themselves were willing to make a contribution. The flood-gates of the past were opened at 'Speak Bitterness' meetings which revealed the reasons for their former oppression and degradation. At the same time they were taught a trade and spent part of the day in productive work for which they were paid at the same rate as other workers. They were free to leave whenever they wished and were encouraged to organize their own committees for study, work and recreation. Those who were illiterate learned to read and write. Those who could sing, dance, act or write plays gave performances in their own centres and in others in different parts of the country. Visits from family members were encouraged. When their rehabilitation was complete, they were either found jobs in the city or returned to their native villages where their economic security was guaranteed. One of them, Lu Shen Li, ex-prostitute from Kiangsu province, wrote a most moving letter in which she said, 'People in different societies have different fates. The old society made people into devils; the new society makes devils into people.'

Now the Rehabilitation Centres have all closed down for there is no further need for them. Some have been converted into factories and among their veteran workers are ex-prostitutes, most of whom have married and some have joined the Communist Party.

The transformation of the position of women

The closure of brothels and legislation outlawing prostitution cannot, of course, be equated with the elimination of prostitution or with the complete emancipation of women. The only fundamental way to do this is first to change the structure of society and then change the thinking of those who comprise it. The first found expression in the Common Programme of the Chinese People's Political Consultative Conference of 1949 and the Marriage Law of 1950 which freed women from feudal bondage and gave them equal rights with men.

Changing the moral values and deep-rooted customs of millions of people takes a very long time and necessitates unremitting effort. Great progress has been made since Liberation and Chinese women are now approaching genuine equality with men. They occupy important posts in every sphere of governmental, political, productive and cultural work, and sex relations based on inequality are disappearing. Although it would be an exaggeration to say that they have already achieved 100 per cent emancipation, it can be confidently stated that history has never before witnessed such a transformation in the status of women as has happened in China since 1949.

The elimination of poverty

Although China is still a poor country, it is possible to talk of the elimination of poverty because poverty is relative and only has meaning in relation to the productive level and social system of a given country at a given time. Certainly a situation such as that quoted above, in which twenty million people were described as being on the verge of starvation and in which an influx of girl slaves and prostitutes into the cities was regarded as inevitable, cannot recur. No one in China is allowed to fall below a subsistence level, to starve, to become homeless or to be without adequate clothing. No one is forced to beg or steal in order to stay alive. No one is burdened down by debt. Millions of new jobs have been created and a widespread system of social security is being built up. A clause in the Constitution reads: 'Working people in the People's Republic of China have the right to material assistance in old age and in case of illness or disability.'

The economic roots of prostitution and crime have been cut for ever.

Mass campaigns against syphilis

The First National Health Conference in August 1950 adopted four guiding principles:

Health work should primarily serve the masses of the labouring people.

Chief emphasis should be placed on the prevention of disease.

Close unity should be fostered between traditional and modern doctors.

Health work should, whenever appropriate, be conducted by mass campaigns with the active participation of medical workers.

In the same year the Ministry of Health organized teams to investigate the venereal disease situation throughout the country and to work out plans for prevention and treatment. The following year an assault on venereal diseases in the National Minority regions was started.

In 1954, the Central Research Institute of Dermatology and Venereology was established to co-ordinate the field work and initiate appropriate research and training programmes.

In 1958, the Research Institute organized pilot projects in eight different provinces and when some initial successes had been scored, the Ministry of Health called a nation-wide conference to study the experience gained in Ningtu county, Kiangsi. Characteristically, the conference was held in the little township where the work had actually been done and where participants could see it with their own eyes, discuss it with the local people and gain first-hand experience of its successes and problems.

Mobilizing an army of fighters against syphilis

To find and treat millions of cases of syphilis and change the attitude of tens of millions of ordinary folk towards venereal disease, the existing corps of medical personnel was totally inadequate. A new approach was needed involving the mobilizing and training of thousands of paramedical workers and immediately a number of highly controversial questions arose. What sort of people should be trained? What minimal educational standards should they possess? How, where and in what should they be trained? Were qualified doctors from the old society able to train others or did they themselves need to learn more before they could teach?

In the course of prolonged and at times heated discussions it gradually became clear that to meet the challenge of eliminating venereal disease from the world's most populous country, the basic necessity was for medical workers to acquire a new philosophy, and a new style of work based on the thinking of Mao Tse-tung.

At the same time, they needed to become familiar with the signs and symptoms of venereal disease, with the technique of blood testing and with methods of treatment.

This combination of political and professional qualifications is in China called becoming 'Red and Expert'.

Once agreement had been reached on these basic principles, it was easy to find the answers to the controversial questions concerning methods of training and recruitment.

As the work progressed, and particularly as the formerly backward Minority regions caught up with the rest of China, the training and composition of medical teams underwent a change. For example, in 1952 when the first medical team went to Inner Mongolia, all its sixty members came from Peking, for there were not yet any modern Mongolian doctors. They lived and worked in yurts, a sort of felt-covered wigwam. In 1962, for the much bigger task of re-surveying the entire population, all but six of the team were Mongolians and they had access to first-class laboratory facilities in the newly-built medical school in Paotow. In 1962, there were 177,418 primary and secondary school students and 2,517 college students in Mongolia whereas, at the time of Liberation, ninety per cent of Mongolians had been illiterate.

The teachers had, for the most part, been trained in the old society as private practitioners and so they, together with the trainees, studied politics and especially the 'Three Old Articles',[1] learned to mix with ordinary people and tried to get rid of their old feelings of conceit and superiority for, as Chairman Mao put it, 'To be a teacher of the people, one must first be a pupil of the people.'

Gradually, on the basis of a common political outlook, unity was established between teachers and pupils, between traditional and modern doctors, between the masses and the whole body of medical and paramedical workers, and this unity was further strengthened during the course of actual work.

New methods of case finding

To find the millions of cases of latent syphilis scattered throughout the country was an immense undertaking which could not be tackled along orthodox lines.

[1] 'In Memory of Norman Bethune.' Mao Tse-tung, *Selected Works*, *Vol. II, p.* 337; 'Serve the People.' Mao Tse-tung, *Selected Works*, *Vol. III, p.* 227; 'The Foolish Old Man Who Removed Mountains.' Mao Tse-tung, *Selected Works*, *Vol. III, p.* 321.

Opinions were divided as to how it could be done. Those with conservative, stereotyped thinking urged greater working efficiency, more personnel, better and speedier methods of blood testing and more expenditure. Theirs was a purely technical approach. Those who could think in a bold, revolutionary way urged a political approach, with reliance on the initiative of the masses as the key to success. The political approach won out, although not without a struggle. . . .

In a county in Hopei province, after prolonged discussions between political and medical workers, a form was drawn up asking ten questions, an affirmative answer to any one of which would suggest the possibility of syphilis. These ten questions contained 'clues' such as a history of a skin rash, falling hair, genital sore or exposure to the risk of infection. To draw up the questionnaire was one thing; to persuade tens of thousands of people to fill it in, honestly and conscientiously, was quite another thing. To do this intensive propaganda and education was carried out by anti-syphilis fighters who were able to make close contact with the people, give them the concept that they should liberate themselves, and enlist them as allies in the struggle. Propaganda posters were put up in the village streets, one-act plays performed in the market place, talks given over the village radio system and meetings, big and small, held night after night at which the purpose of the questionnaire was explained and the co-operation of the peasants gradually won. The opening talk would be brief and to-the-point and would go something like this: 'Comrades, syphilis is a disease that was bequeathed to us by the rotten society we have thrown out. It's no fault of yours if you have syphilis and no shame should be attached to it. It's only shameful if you cling to your syphilis when you can easily get rid of it. We've got rid of the landlords and the blood-sucking government that looked after *their* interests and now we have a government that looks after *ours*. We have a Party that speaks for us and shows us how to go forward. Now it calls on us to get rid of syphilis and we should seize the opportunity. This form asks ten questions and you should answer them honestly. We will be glad to help any of you who can't read or write. If you don't remember the answers to some of the questions, ask your friends and relatives. In fact, there's nothing wrong with friends and relatives jogging your memories even when they're not asked. This is *our* country now and we should all be concerned about the well-being of everyone else.

'Comrades, we're going forward to Communism and we can't take this rotten disease with us.'

At first in some places the response was slow; few villagers filled in the questionnaire and some of those who did so, concealed one or other of the 'clues'. More propaganda was done and more meetings were called at which the main speakers were those who had already been diagnosed as having syphilis and had been cured by a few injections. They told of the mental struggles they had gone through before admitting to the clues, and of their feelings after they had been cured. They recalled the brutality and indifference of the old days and contrasted it with the present.

The trickle of diagnosed cases increased until it became a torrent. News of the questionnaire, spread by political workers, attracted peasants from far and wide who came to the treatment centres eager to be diagnosed and treated.

All those having clues were given a blood test and it was found that one in twenty of them actually had syphilis. This reduced the problem of case finding to manageable proportions, but the sceptics were not convinced. They said this method was too crude, that it was not scientific, that politics couldn't diagnose syphilis, that it wasn't known how many cases had been missed. Accordingly, the Research Institute decided to test the method, improved in the light of experience, in Ningtu county, Kiangsi province, where the VD rate was known to be high.

The People's Communes assembled three thousand volunteers, some of whom, after suitable study, were given the political task of mobilizing the people to regard the fight against syphilis as their own fight. The remainder were given a seven-day course on the principles of diagnosis and treatment, at the end of which they examined some 3,000 people under the scrutiny of experts, who checked on their results, questioned them, and watched them perform blood tests. Eighty per cent of the trainees passed this stringent practical and theoretical examination and thereby qualified to work independently. One old professor, who had been particularly sceptical, examined a trainee for twenty minutes without getting a wrong answer to his probing questions. He then graciously expressed his complete approval in the classical Chinese phrase, 'I bow to the ground with all the five points of my body.'

The campaign went on for two months, covering not only syphilis, but also such diseases as ringworm of the scalp, leprosy and malaria. Forty-nine thousand cases were examined and treated.

Then the results were checked. Some 30,000 people who had been 'processed' by the trainees on the basis of the questionnaire were given a full clinical and serological examination by qualified doctors. It was found that 90·2 per cent of all sufferers from venereal disease had been discovered.

The value of the mass line method had been conclusively proved and the baffling problem of finding one case in a hundred or one case in a thousand among 500 million peasants had been solved.

In the National Minority areas, this method was not suitable and total population surveys were carried out.

In the cities, several case-finding methods were used including examination of selected age groups, of service trade groups, of army entrants, of those about to marry, of pregnant women and of residents in particular lanes and localities. In some cities, the whole population was covered; in others, only those sections who were particularly at risk. In Shanghai, where the VD rate at the time of Liberation was as high as five per cent, the whole population was tested and to do this some 3,600 technicians were trained to perform the rapid fresh blood slide test for syphilis, which gives an answer of ninety-two per cent accuracy within twenty minutes and which requires only two drops of blood from a prick in the ear.

Active treatment

Once the sufferers from syphilis had been discovered, treatment was a relatively simple matter although this, too, aroused some controversy around the question as to whether or not trainees with little knowledge and experience should be allowed to give treatment. Some elderly doctors with a strong 'closed-shop' mentality, argued that it would be unethical and unwise to allow such people to carry out treatment. But the Ningtu experience refuted their arguments and, moreover, it was obvious that for many years to come there would not be enough fully qualified doctors to carry the work load.

Penicillin was proved to be superior to all other forms of treatment and Chinese antibiotic factories were by now producing enough to supply all domestic needs, leaving a surplus for sending to impoverished newly-emerging nations.

Criteria of cure

The new approach to syphilis demanded a concept of cure which extended beyond the individual to include the whole community. The criteria for community cure were strict. They included the finding and treatment of all existing cases, a total absence of new cases appearing in the community, disappearance of congenital syphilis in new-born babies, and normal pregnancies and pregnancy outcomes in previously treated mothers. When these criteria had been fulfilled and maintained for five years, the community was considered to be cured. This has already been achieved in most areas and soon, with continued follow-up measures to detect the rare case of recurrent or congenital syphilis, it will undoubtedly be reached throughout the country.

That is how China, once the so-called 'sick man of Asia', became the first country in the world to conquer syphilis.

10

Death to the snails!
The fight against schistosomiasis

What is schistosomiasis?

One of the world's greatest scourges, schistosomiasis affects some 250 million people in Africa, Asia, Asia Minor, Central and South America, and claims a vast toll in death and suffering.

Because it is one of the most difficult diseases to eradicate, it is sometimes called the 'Unconquerable Disease'.

By using a combined medical and political approach, similar to that employed in the eradication of syphilis, it seems likely that China will be the first country in the world to bring this disease under effective control.

On a world scale, there are three main varieties of schistosomiasis which are similar in essentials while differing in details. The following description applies to Schistosomiasis Japonicum, the form which is widespread in the Far East and the form most resistant to treatment. The disease is caused by a blood fluke or microscopic worm which inhabits the blood-vessels of the liver and intestines. The female, about half an inch long and the thickness of a strand of fine wool, lives in a groove on the undersurface of the thicker and shorter male. The pair of worms travel against the blood-stream until they lodge in a fine blood-vessel in the wall of the intestine where the female lays up to a hundred eggs, some of which are swept back into the liver while others remain in the wall of the intestine. The eggs then escape from the blood-vessels and cause chronic inflammation of the liver and intestine.

Symptoms

Intestinal inflammation and ulceration cause bleeding, anaemia, malnutrition and sometimes intestinal obstruction or perforation. Chronic liver inflammation causes hardening of the liver which obstructs the flow of blood from the stomach and intestine, and results in the outpouring of large quantities of fluid into the abdominal cavity and sometimes in severe haemorrhage into the stomach.

The belly becomes distended, partly by fluid and partly by the spleen, which may enlarge until it weighs as much as twenty pounds instead of its normal seven to eight ounces.

Children fail to develop both in height and sexually; women cease to menstruate and men become incapable of parenthood. Thus the death rate increases while the birth rate decreases giving rise to serious depopulation.

The life cycle of the blood fluke

The eggs which penetrate the wall of the intestine are passed in the faeces and if they come into contact with water they develop into free-swimming larvae. These search for the intermediate host, an amphibious snail of genus *oncomelania* having a screw-type shell less than $\frac{1}{4}$ inch in length, within which the larvae multiply into immature flukes or *cercariae* which are discharged in huge numbers during the daylight hours—usually between 9 a.m. and 2 p.m. As many as 1,000 *cercariae* may be discharged daily from a single snail. They have forked tails, can swim vigorously and if one of them finds its way to a suitable warm-blooded host, such as man, it sheds its tail and by using a complicated system of glands and 'grappling hooks', burrows through the skin and penetrates into a blood-vessel. Here it develops into its adult form, and repeats its life cycle.

THE PREVENTION OF SCHISTOSOMIASIS

Theoretically, schistosomiasis can be prevented by interrupting the life cycle of the blood fluke at three points.

One is to prevent the host from coming into contact with water containing the free-swimming *cercariae* for these could not develop and multiply if they did not find refuge in blood-vessels.

The second is to prevent faeces containing live eggs from contaminating river water where the eggs can hatch into larvae.

The third is by attacking the intermediate hosts, the snails, for if these were eliminated, the larvae could not develop into *cercariae*.

In the fight against schistosomiasis, all three points in the life cycle of the blood fluke are attacked, but since they are not equally vulnerable, they are not attacked with equal force.

Schistosomiasis in China occurs mostly in the lower Yangtze valley where, as recently as 1955, there were estimated to be more than ten million sufferers. The area is dotted with lakes and criss-crossed by canals and rivers. Rice cultivation predominates and, since rice is transplanted under water, it is nearly impossible for farmers to avoid contact with potentially infected water. Moreover, there are hundreds of thousands of boatmen, fishermen and irrigation workers who inevitably come into contact with river and canal water. It is, therefore, difficult to break the cycle at the point where the *cercariae* penetrate the skin of the host, but if rice transplantation and cultivation could be mechanized, and some progress is being made in this direction, contact with infected water could be greatly reduced. Barrier creams and lotions which repel the *cercariae* as they approach the body are being tried out. Rubber boots and gloves have been used, but they have many disadvantages. Swimming in infected waterways is strongly discouraged and the people are urged to wash clothes and dishes in safe well-water rather than in contaminated river water.

However, the main emphasis in prevention is on the other two points in the cycle.

Contamination of waterways with infected faeces could, of course, be prevented by curing all infected persons. This method would be ideal, but, for many reasons, it would be unrealistic to place excessive reliance on it. Late cases, which cannot readily be cured, are a constant source of eggs. Not all sufferers can be diagnosed and treated at the same time, for this is a disease involving millions of people and huge areas. Even if this could be done, oxen, cattle, buffaloes, rats and dogs, which are all susceptible to schistosomiasis, would still contaminate the waterways and cause reinfection of those already cured.

The best method of preventing contamination of waterways is to treat all human faeces so as to kill the eggs of schistosomiasis, for in China human excrement is indispensable as a soil fertilizer.

This can be done by storing excrement for fifteen to twenty days before use, so that it generates enough ammonia and heat to kill the harmful parasites. One method of storage is in concrete tanks having three compartments separated by controllable barriers. Fresh night soil is accumulated in the first compartment from which it is transferred at intervals to the second compartment where it remains for fifteen days. Then, safe for use, it flows into the third compartment from which it is taken as required.

The manure of oxen and cattle is treated in the same way.

MAN AGAINST SNAILS

The prevention of schistosomiasis at the third point in the cycle, by striking at the snails, the intermediate host, is the most laborious but nevertheless the most promising point of attack, for if snails could be eliminated, schistosomiasis would disappear.

A gigantic campaign against snails was therefore launched.

First the habits of the snails were intensively studied and it was found that they are most abundant close to the waterline, especially in dark places, that they can burrow into the mud for a depth of three inches, that they can migrate ten yards in one year, that their life-span is about five years and that they quickly die if they are deprived of water or air.

On the basis of this knowledge, a grand strategy for the elimination of snails by temporarily draining all infected waterways and removing and burying the snail-containing layers from their sides was worked out.

This was where politics and preventive medicine merged, with politics in the leading position, for the scheme was so huge in its scope, that it could not possibly succeed without the leadership of the Party, without the fullest and most active support from millions of people and without a correct overall strategic plan.

The strategy which was adopted was a result of the living study and living application of three major concepts which had been worked out by Mao Tse-tung and repeatedly tested in practice during the long revolutionary wars.

The Mass Line

The first concept rests on the conviction that the ordinary people possess great strength and wisdom and that when their initiative is given full play they can accomplish miracles; that the art of leadership is to learn from the masses, to refine and systematize their experience and, on this basis, to decide on policy.

To mobilize the peasantry against the snails, it was first necessary to explain to them the nature of the illness which had plagued them for so long and for this purpose lectures, film shows, posters, radio-talks were employed. When the peasants came to understand the nature of their enemy, they themselves worked out methods of defeating it.

Twice a year, in March and in August, the entire population in county after county, supplemented by the voluntary labour of all available armymen,

96

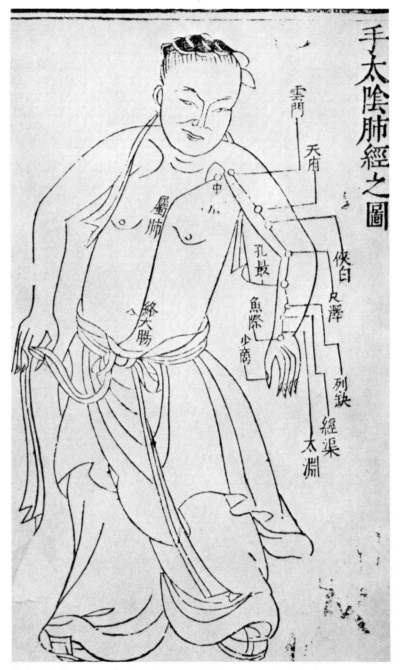

手太陰肺經之圖

雲門

天府

中府

屬肺

俠白

孔最

尺澤

魚際

少商

絡大腸

列缺

經渠

太淵

A drawing from an early eleventh-century Chinese manuscript showing acupuncture points on the body. *Bibliotheque Nationale, Paris*

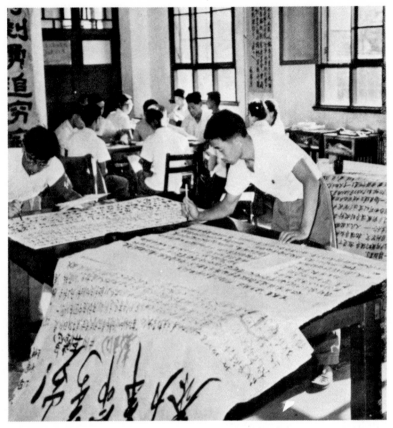

Cultural Revolution. Above: school students writing Big-Character Posters.

Opposite: similar Posters in a Shanghai street and a Kiangsu village.

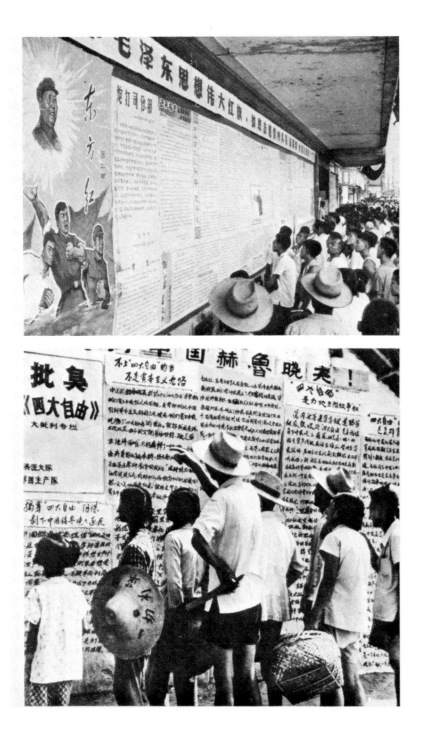

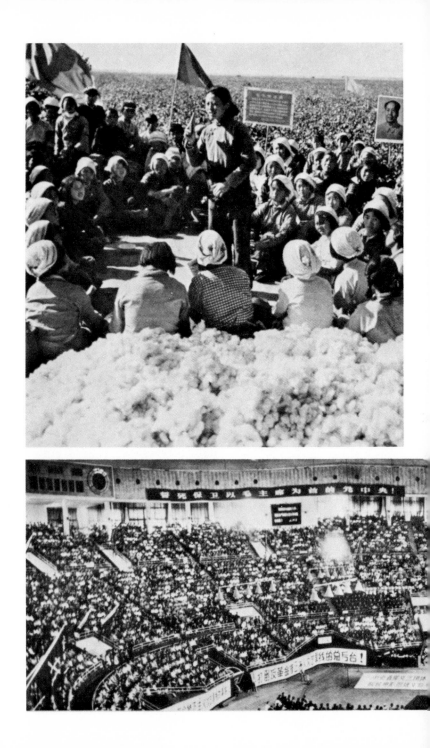

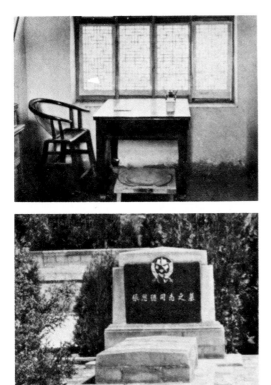

Far left and below: two aspects of the Cultural Revolution, a lunch-break meeting in a Shantung cotton field, and a mass meeting in a Peking stadium.

This page, above: the cave in Yenan where Chairman Mao lived and where he wrote some of his best-known works. Below: the grave of Chang Szu-teh in Yenan where, on 8 September 1944, at a memorial meeting for Chang Szu-teh, Mao Tse-tung delivered his famous speech 'Serve the People'.

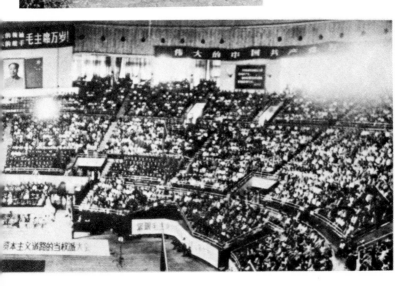

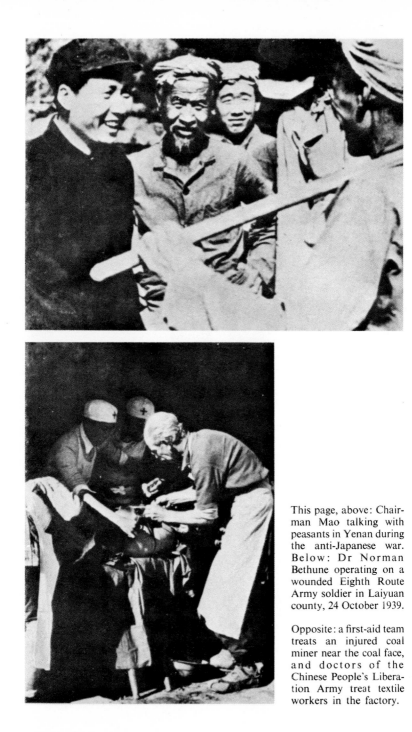

This page, above: Chairman Mao talking with peasants in Yenan during the anti-Japanese war. Below: Dr Norman Bethune operating on a wounded Eighth Route Army soldier in Laiyuan county, 24 October 1939.

Opposite: a first-aid team treats an injured coal miner near the coal face, and doctors of the Chinese People's Liberation Army treat textile workers in the factory.

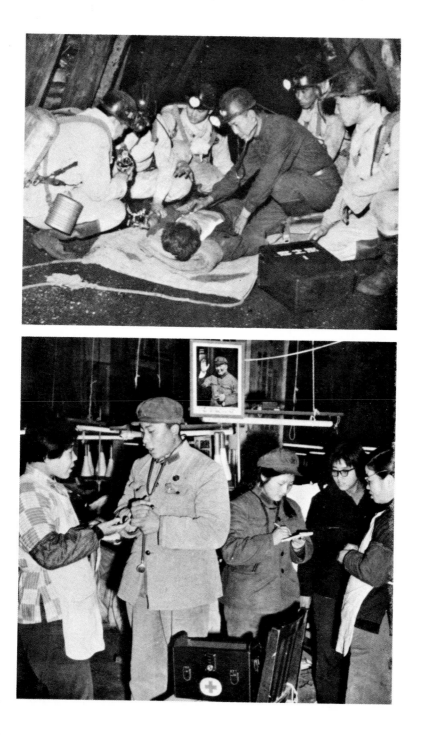

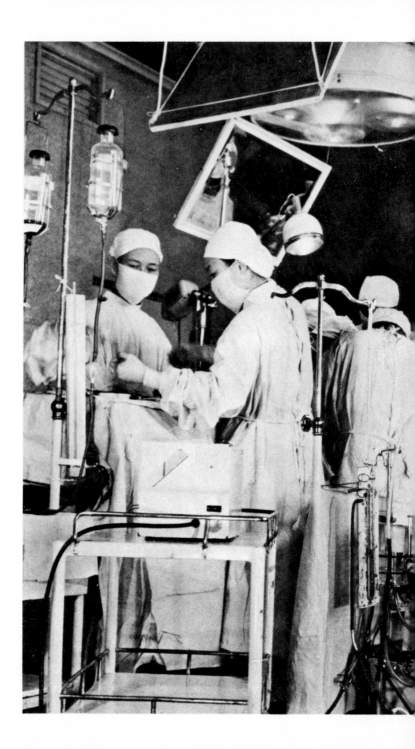

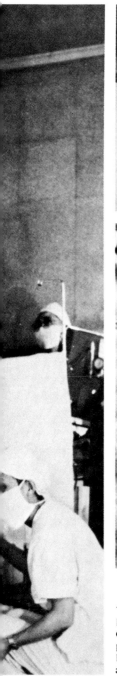

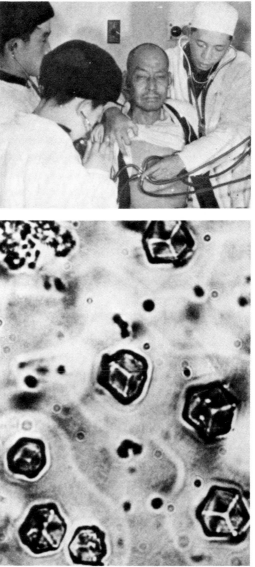

Three aspects of Chinese medical progress. Left: a heart operation in progress. In the foreground is a Chinese-made heart-lung apparatus. Above, top: peasant doctors attend a refresher course in Peking. Below: a microscopic view of synthetic, biologically active, crystalline insulin.

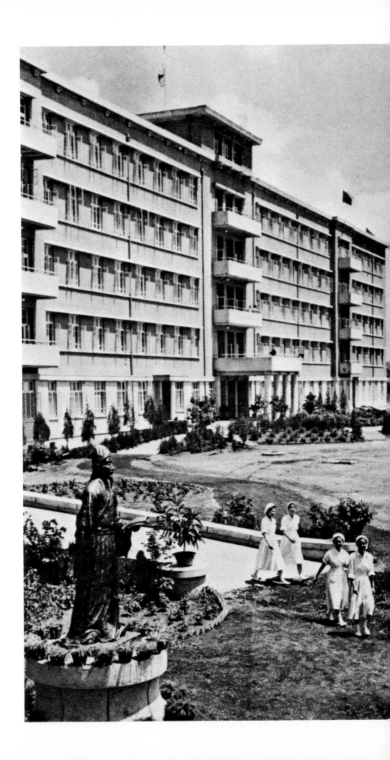

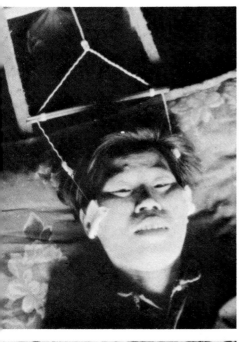

Medicine in the capital and in the countryside.

Opposite: the Third Hospital attached to Peking Medical College. The statue is of the Ming dynasty pharmacologist Li Shi-chen.

This page, above: the soldier's wife (see chapter 14) undergoing improvised head traction for dislocation of the neck with injury of the spinal cord. Below: the soldier's wife, a few months later, fully recovered.

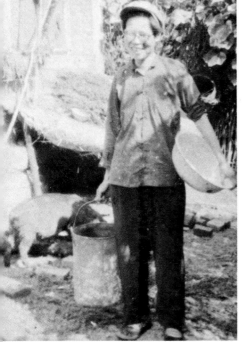

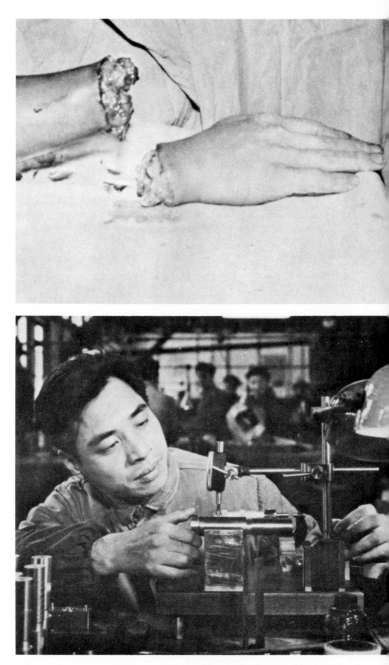

Above: the severed right hand of Shanghai worker Wang Cung-po. Below: Wa Cung-po at work three years after reattachment of his severed hand.

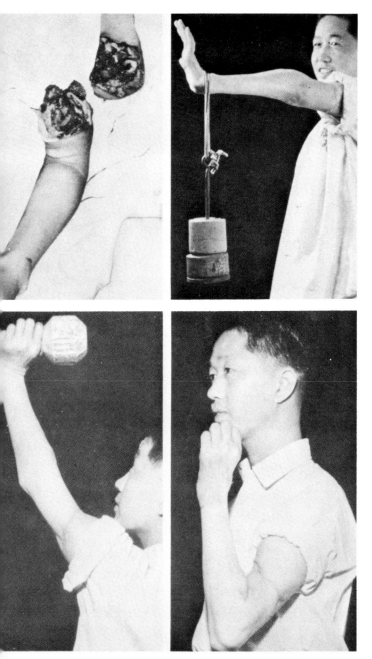

ve: left arm severed above the elbow, and the same patient exercising after
achment of the limb.

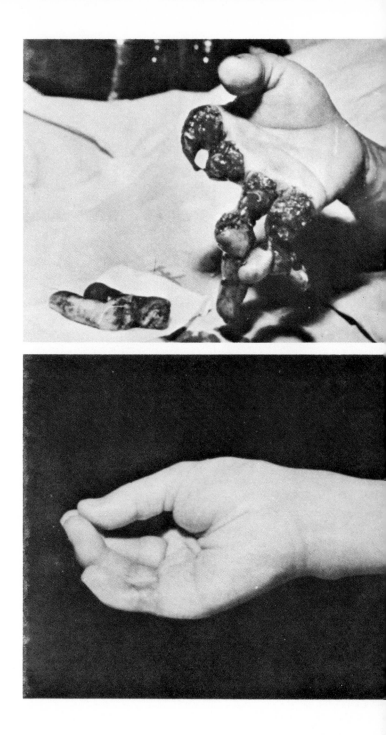

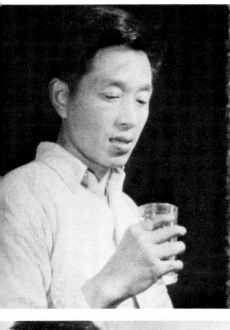

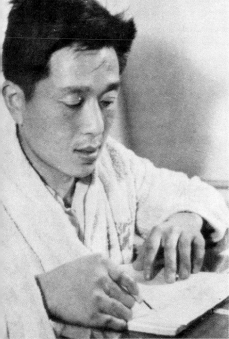

A case of multiple finger amputations, and the patient demonstrating that, after reattachment, he can use his hand almost normally.

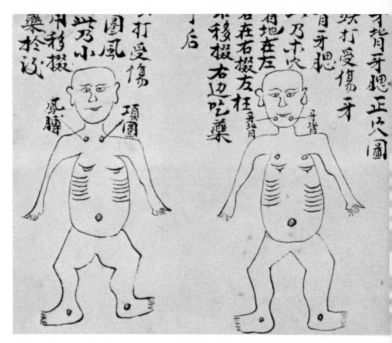

A drawing showing the pressure points for use in manipulation, from a manuscript of the early eighteenth century containing prescriptions for various diseases. *Wellcome Foundation, London*

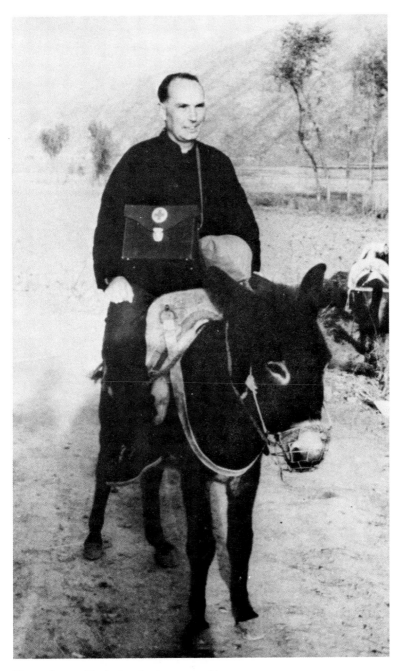

The author on his donkey in the countryside.

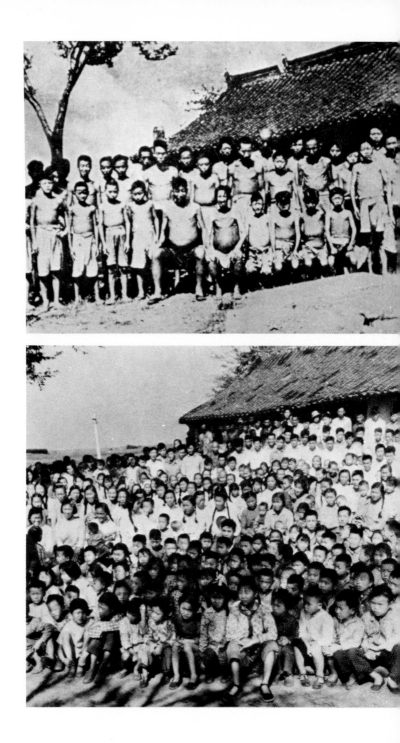

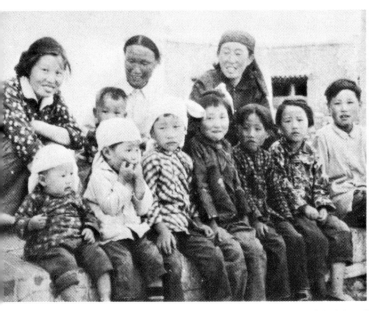

ove: a formerly childless Mongolian woman (in black headscarf) with eight of nine children, after being cured of syphilis.

e two pictures on the left were taken in Ren Tun village, Ching Pu county. The one was taken soon after Liberation, when nearly all the villagers suffered from istosomiasis. The lower one was taken at the same spot in 'the village that came ife', after schistosomiasis had been practically eliminated.

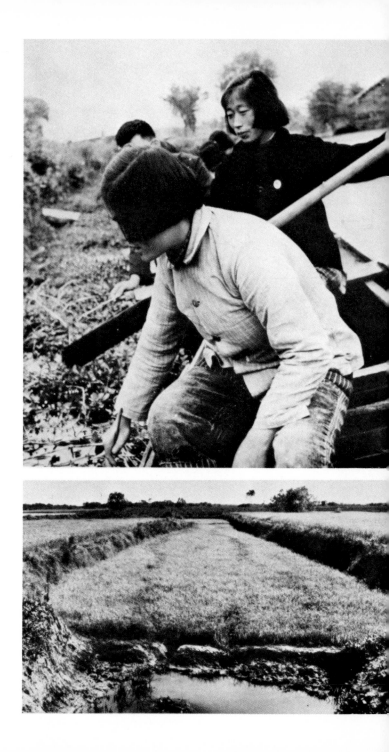

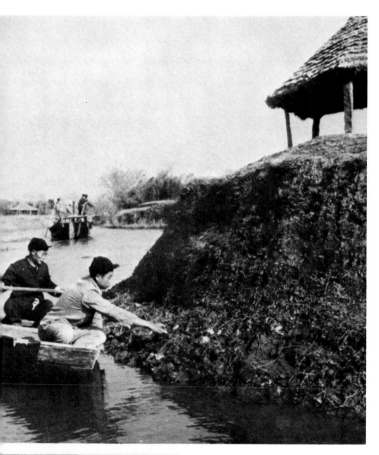

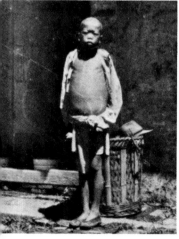

Above, left and right: searching the river banks for schistosomiasis-carrying snails.

Opposite: a snail-infested waterway in Ren Tun village after it had been filled and planted with rice.

Left: an advanced case of schistosomiasis, showing under-development, emaciation and severe abdominal distension.

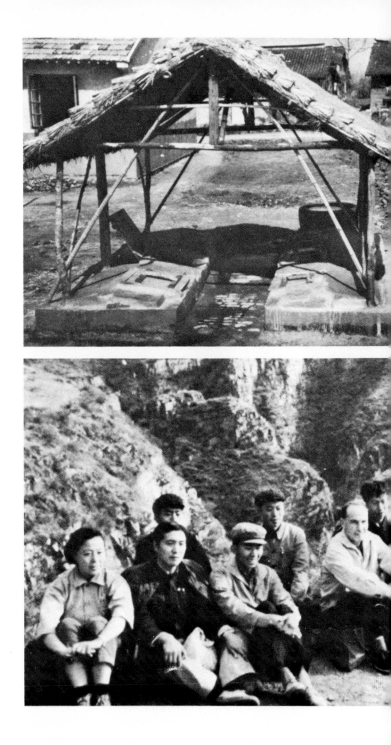

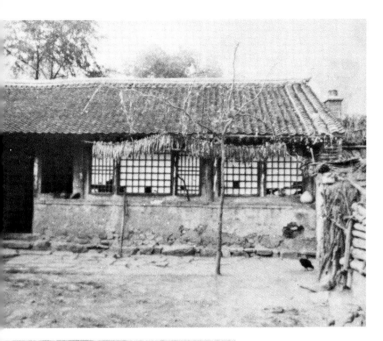

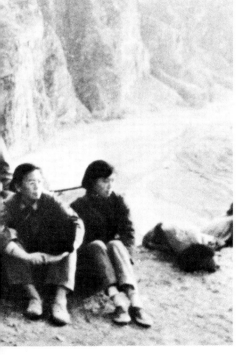

Left: a mobile medical team, including the author, resting on a mountain path, and, above, one of the hygienic village latrines which they constructed.

Above, right: the cottage in which Fragrant Lotus was delivered of her child (see chapter 15).

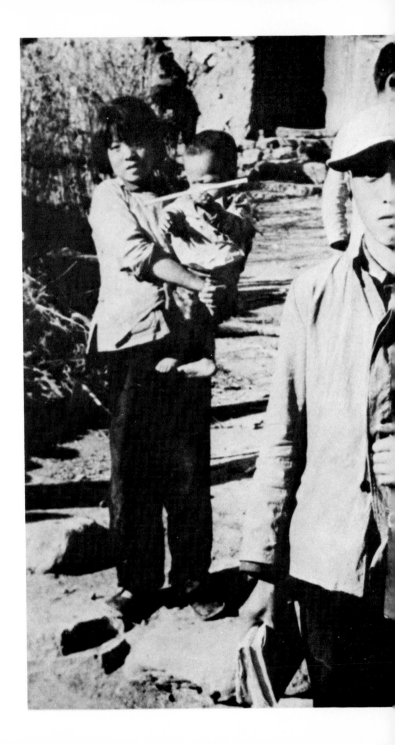

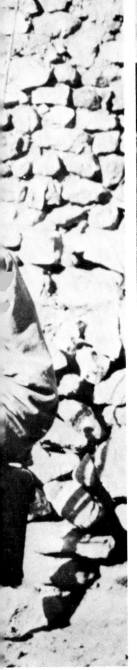

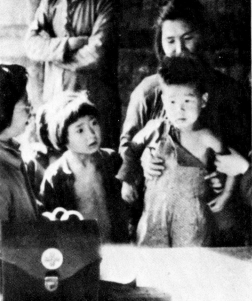

Left: Wang Sheng-li, a
peasant doctor, on his
rounds.

Above: a village inocula-
tion team at work.

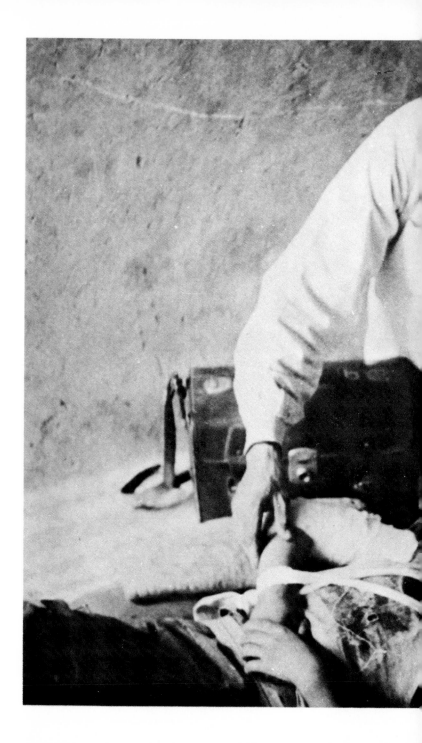

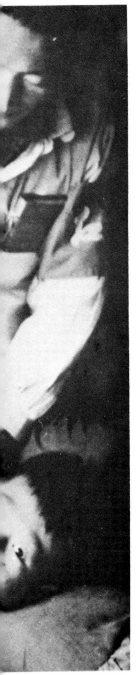

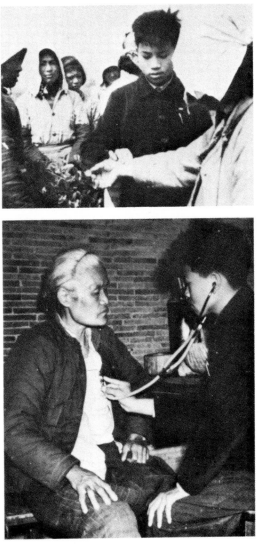

Peasant doctors at work.

Left: a small boy's broken arm is set on the kang in his own cottage.

This page: a woman is treated while she works in the fields, and another undergoes a medical examination in her cottage.

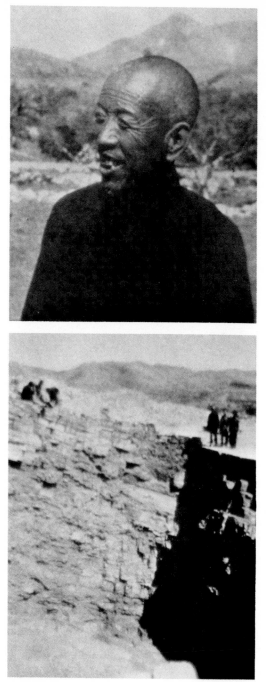

This page, above: Old Zhang of the 'Three-legged Donkey' production brigade (see chapter 5). Below: the irrigation cistern hewn out of living rock at the 'Three-legged Donkey' production brigade. It was while working on this that Old Zhang sustained his injury. A few minutes after this photograph was taken, the cistern started to fill with water.

Opposite, above: terracing in what was originally the 'Three-legged Donkey Co-op'. Below: the lame donkey, now pensioned off, which inspired the name of the production brigade. The board displays quotations from the writings of Chairman Mao.

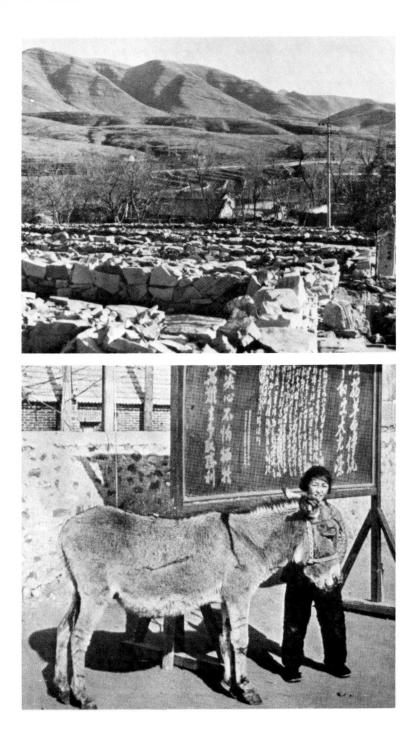

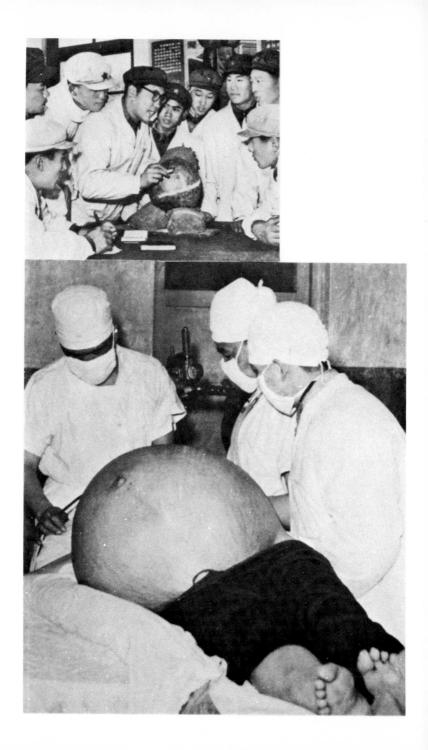

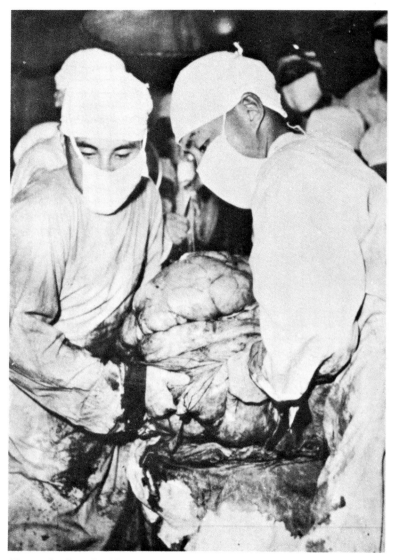

Above: the forty-five-kilogramme tumour being carried away from the operating table at the conclusion of the operation on peasant woman Chang Chiu-chu (described by the author in 'Postscript').

Opposite, below: a photograph taken just before the operation commenced. Above: armymen discuss the incision. One of them is sketching his proposal on a gourd.

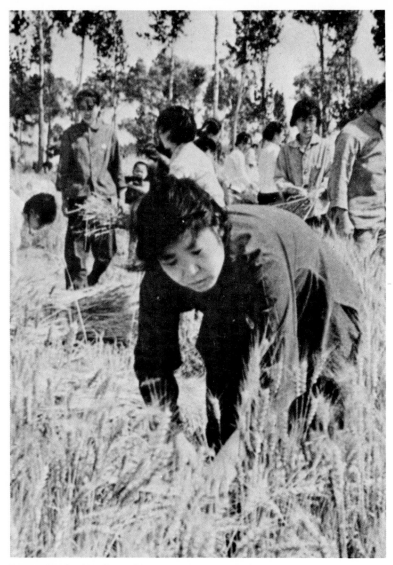

Restored to health, Chang Chiu-chu helps in harvesting the wheat.

students, teachers and office workers, turned out to drain the rivers and ditches, dig away and bury their banks and tamp down the buried earth.

To empty a complicated system of water channels demands more than back-breaking work; it also requires careful planning for if they are emptied out of proper sequence, serious waterlogging may result. Reliance on the knowledge of the peasants is of key importance. To mobilize the masses does not mean to issue them with shovels and instructions; it means to fire them with enthusiasm, to release their initiative and to tap their wisdom.

Concentration of forces

The second concept in the fight against the snails was that of concentrating a superior force to win battles of annihilation.

At a time when the People's Liberation Army was heavily outnumbered by its enemies and grossly inferior in terms of weapons, Mao Tse-tung summarized a set of military tactics which, within two years, helped to win nation-wide victory. One of them was—'In every battle, concentrate an absolutely superior force, encircle the enemy forces completely, strive to wipe them out thoroughly and do not let any escape from the net.'[1]

This tactic was applied in the battle against the snails by selecting focal points for decisive attack. Of the ten infected counties around Shanghai, two were selected as the main targets in the early stages of what was to be a prolonged campaign. All available labour power, medical resources, pumps, river-draining and damming equipment were concentrated in these two counties and, within a short time, the snails there had suffered a mortal blow. Then the forces were re-grouped and the attack was directed elsewhere. Gradually, extensive snail-free zones were created.

The Paper Tiger theory

The third concept was that embodied in the famous 'Paper Tiger' theory which is often misrepresented in the West.

Mao first used the term 'Paper Tiger' in 1946 to describe the formidable USA/Kuomintang combination which so heavily outnumbered and out-gunned the Communist armies, and some years later, when history had brilliantly confirmed his theory, he further elaborated it:

'Just as there is not a single thing in the world without a dual nature (this is the law of the unity of opposites), so imperialism and all reactionaries have a dual nature—they are real tigers and paper tigers at the same time. . . . On the one hand, they are real tigers; they devoured people, devoured people by the millions and tens of millions. . . . But in the end they changed into paper tigers, dead tigers, bean-curd tigers. . . . Hence, imperialism and all reactionaries, looked at in essence, from a long-term point of view, from a strategic point of view, must be seen for what they are—paper tigers. On this we should build our strategic thinking. On the other hand, they are also living tigers, iron tigers, real tigers which can devour people. On this we should build our tactical thinking.'[2]

[1] 'The Present Situation and Our Tasks'. 25 December, 1947; *Selected Military Writings*, 2nd ed., pp. 349-50.

[2] Speech at meeting of Political Bureau of Central Committee of C.C.P. held in Wuchang on 1 December, 1958, quoted in *Selected Works, Vol. IV, pp.* 98-99.

Thus, the 'Paper Tiger' theory is not a simple black-and-white proposition for 'Paper Tigers' are both paperish and tigerish. Applied to the fight against snails it means, on the one hand, that since the snails are harmful to mankind, no matter how numerous, well camouflaged and well protected they are, in the long run they are doomed because man is incomparably more powerful and will eventually solve this problem.

On the other hand, it means that although the snails are doomed they are a formidable opponent that must be taken seriously. No complacency is permissible; every battle must be planned down to the last detail; all weapons brought into play.

The strategic concept of confidence in final victory found expression in the response of millions of peasants which made possible an unprecedented mobilization of manpower and resources. The tactical concept of taking the enemy seriously found expression in well-planned, versatile methods of attack and constant vigilance. For example, if the sides of the waterways are so covered by reeds or other plants that snails can find refuge among them, flame throwers are used to burn down the vegetation and scorch the banks. Under bridges, or if a waterway cannot be completely drained, poisonous chemicals like Sodium Pentachlorophenate or Calcium Cyanamide are used to destroy the snails.

In between large-scale campaigns, regular anti-snail patrols are maintained by trained snail-spotters who cruise along the rivers in canoes, scrutinizing the banks for snails. I spent many hours with such a team in the spring of 1967 and although we never found a live snail, they intend to continue a daily search. I asked the leader of the team, a young woman who had herself suffered from schistosomiasis, whether she found the work boring. 'Yes,' she said. 'It can be very boring and trying. On hot days I get scorched and my head aches. Mosquitoes buzz around and under bridges, and in the dark places where we have to search most carefully, there are all sorts of creepy-crawly things. The children, too, used to annoy us. At first they didn't understand what we were doing and they used to walk along the bank laughing at us and asking us why we didn't do proper work like the other grown-ups instead of playing about in boats all day. I sometimes felt like asking to be transferred to ordinary agricultural work, but then I remembered how I had felt when I suffered from schistosomiasis as a child and I decided to carry on with this work, for a life-time if necessary. We asked some of the children to come with us in the canoe and after they experienced the discomforts themselves, they soon stopped jeering at us.'

CASE-FINDING

Prevention comes first but treatment is also important and the first step in treatment is case-finding, which is mainly done by examination of faeces. I visited a faeces examination station in a derelict temple staffed by a young girl Commune member, an old man who had asked to be allowed to do this job when arthritis of the knees prevented him from working in the fields, and by Doctor Chu, a cheerful young man with a deeply suntanned face, gleaming teeth and untidy hair. Dr Chu had studied medicine for barely three years but what he lacked in book knowledge he made up for in common sense, organizing ability and enthusiasm. He had set up a series of faeces testing stations throughout the Commune, had trained the staff for them and visited them regularly to check up and compile the statistics. The young girl did most of the talking. 'We test the faeces of everybody in our area twice a year and the main difficulty is to persuade people to send in specimens. They sometimes regard it as a great joke and play tricks on us. For reliability we like to test three different specimens, but, though we explained this very clearly, some people play dumb, divide one stool into three parts and send them in one after another. Others try to fool us by sending us dog or ox dung. Old Chen here,' she said, indicating her arthritic companion, 'chases up these Smart-Alecs and gives them a lecture and then they nearly always send in their specimens.'

'I don't give lectures,' said Old Chen. 'I'm no good at lecturing. I just tell them what it used to be like here in the old days when practically everybody had a big belly and they soon see the point.'

Dr Chu showed me the process of testing faeces. A small quantity of faeces is put into a conical flask which is filled with water, stirred and allowed to sediment. The supernatant fluid is then poured off and the process is repeated three times so as to reduce the amount of debris in the faeces and make it easier to identify eggs. The sediment is then examined under a microscope. If no eggs are found, a hatching test is carried out. A piece of faeces is placed in a flask, covered with water and kept in a hot dark room. If eggs are present, they hatch into larvae which rise to the surface and can be seen as thread-like structures which all point in the same direction when a light is thrown on them.

The aim is to examine the faeces of everyone in the endemic area twice a year. In 1965, 1,300,000 peasants around Shanghai had their faeces tested and seventeen per cent were found to be positive. In 1966, the percentage of positive tests had fallen to twelve per cent, many of whom had either relapsed after a course of treatment or were late, resistant cases, while only a small proportion were genuine new infections.

Case-finding on this enormous scale is only possible if simple improvised methods are used and if the people are mobilized to do the job themselves, relying on their own resources rather than on experts from outside.

TREATMENT

Treatment is the weak link in the fight against schistosomiasis.

The most effective drug, antimony tartrate, has a number of drawbacks since it is toxic, causes unpleasant side effects in some patients and has to be given by intravenous injection over a rather prolonged course. To overcome these disadvantages, Chinese scientists have developed a drug which, since it can be taken by mouth, is much more suitable for use in the countryside. However, its efficacy is lower than that of the intravenous drug and it produces delayed toxic reactions in a small but significant proportion of cases. In cases with ascites (fluid in the abdomen) a combination of a traditional herbal drug with the orthodox antimony treatment has many advantages.

In late cases drug therapy alone cannot be relied on to produce a cure and, if the spleen is enlarged or excessively active, its surgical removal may be indicated. I attended such an operation in a little county hospital of sixty

99

beds where 555 operations for removal of the spleen have been performed since it opened in 1958. It is staffed both by local personnel and by specialists from Shanghai, there on rotation.

In spite of the somewhat primitive conditions, I have seldom seen an operation more beautifully performed. Anaesthesia was of the most modern type—high, continuous epidural block which leaves the patient fully conscious, produces complete muscular relaxation and is free from the risks of spinal anaesthesia. The operation was completed in forty minutes and scarcely a teaspoonful of blood was lost from beginning to end.

Removing the spleen in suitable cases has many advantages. Growth in young people is stimulated (one boy grew three inches within four months of the operation); the menstrual periods return and women regain their fertility; the appetite improves; the abdominal swelling gets less; anaemia is corrected and the overall strength and nutritional state improves. Some patients who are too weak to withstand a course of medical treatment, can do so after removal of the spleen.

Other surgical procedures used in treating late cases of schistosomiasis include operations for the relief of intestinal obstruction and for the effects of hardening of the liver.

DIVISIONAL HEADQUARTERS

In order to learn more about the planning and organization behind the huge anti-schistosomiasis campaign, I spent a day in the Schistosomiasis Prevention Station for Ching Pu county. Comrade Chang Kai, in charge of the station, walked with me round the county town which, at first glance, seemed so ancient and archaic that it conjured up a picture of the distant days of Sung or Tang. . . . Cobbled streets so narrow that a horseman would have to squeeze his horse tight if he were not to graze his legs on the houses crowding in on either side; a maze of canals and rivulets spanned by bridges ranging from wooden planks lashed together with rice-straw rope to lion-flanked, hump-backed bridges of hewn stone, marvels of engineering in their day and age but curiously incongruous in the twentieth century; soaring pagodas built according to strict rules, seven or thirteen stories high, no more, no less; a jumble of shops and dwellings, close-packed, where trade, production and the intimacies of everyday life jostled each other for elbow room; boats on the waterways, high prowed, built of thick wood, heavy laden with the produce of the land, a single oarsman straining in the stern.

But if a first glance suggested that nothing had changed, a second would show the profound changes in the underlying essence. Now, the hexagonal pagodas blazon forth political slogans written in huge red characters, slogans unknown in days when the illiterate multitude served the literate few. In the shops, no bartering, no private trade; now no man works for his own profit but only for the good of the collective. In the streets, no silk-clad officials borne by sweating serfs, no whips, no curses, no flamboyant luxury and no grinding poverty. No smells, no piles of dung or refuse; now the people know that filth breeds flies and flies spread disease. Even the rivers have changed; their flanks are smooth with lime or concrete and others, as Chang Kai pointed out, have been filled in to make new thoroughfares wide enough to take the rubber-tyred carts and the proud puffing tractors that go from farm to farm.

We entered divisional headquarters through a cool courtyard and went to an upper room, the walls covered with charts and maps. Comrade Chang spread out his books and ledgers and told me how the fight was going:

'There are twenty-one People's Communes in this county, 620,000 mu of cultivated land and 350,000 people. The whole area is endemic with schistosomiasis. We reckon that at the time of Liberation at least eighty per cent of all able-bodied peasants must have had the disease.

'From Liberation till the end of 1966, we treated 245,000 patients including re-infections and relapses. We have removed 2,276 spleens. We know of 32,000 persons in the county who still excrete schistosomiasis eggs in their faeces; their night-soil is under specially strict supervision.

'The fight against schistosomiasis has gone through four stages.

'In the first stage, before 1955, we mainly reconnoitred. We found that Ching Pu county had 3,500 waterways with snails along 4,300,000 metres of river bank, and in 80,000 mu of rice paddies. At this stage we didn't yet have the concept of relying on the masses. We relied on a few experts from Shanghai and on trained technical personnel working under them. Consequently the work progressed very slowly and the disease continued to wreak havoc.

'The second stage was from 1956-1959. In 1956 agricultural co-operatives were set up throughout China, in 1958, during the Great Leap Forward, they were superseded by the People's Communes and then we really learnt the importance of relying on and mobilizing the masses. The Party drew up the charter for agriculture and one of its forty points was the fight against schistosomiasis. The masses fought against the snails and the infected area gradually shrank. In 1958 alone we treated 80,000 cases, more than in any year before or since.

'The third stage was during the three hard years when natural calamities swept the country and the Soviet revisionists tried to bring us to our knees by disrupting our industrialization.

'Reactionaries at home seized the opportunity to try to negate our achievements, discredit the leadership of Mao Tse-tung and spread confusion and defeatism. It was a period of struggle between those who wanted to advance along the socialist road and those who wanted to call a halt or even return to capitalism. This struggle even showed itself in the fight against schistosomiasis. The reactionaries attacked everything that was new and specifically socialist in our campaign. They poured cold water on the enthusiasm of the masses; they one-sidedly emphasized the importance of experts and equipment; they preached caution and "slow but steady progress"; they derided all our innovations and put forward false slogans such as "do not neglect the towns" at a time when the towns were getting the lion's share of what medical services were available. By advocating more attention to private plots and urging families to use their night-soil on their own plots, they sabotaged our efforts to make night-soil safe. They pretended that they wanted to increase the yield of grain but actually they hated socialism and collective farming.

'During those years the snails were given a respite and they multiplied.

'The fourth and present stage started when our economy had recovered.

101

Since then, Chairman Mao's thinking has increasingly guided our actions and, as a result, we have won great victories in the fight against schistosomiasis. Night-soil control is now in force in 2,584 production teams throughout the county, and more than 6,000 sanitary workers and 331 peasant doctors have been trained. Hospital beds have increased from 40 at the time of Liberation to 565, not including 250 beds in Commune clinics. The length of snail infected river banks has been reduced from 4,300,000 metres to 65,000 metres. and infected paddy fields from 80,000 mu to 6,200 mu. In September and October, 1965, 300,000 man-workdays were spent on snail elimination. In this town, which used to swarm with snails, we couldn't find a single live snail last year. But although we've won some big victories, we have by no means won the final victory. That it still a long way off.'

I expressed my admiration for their achievements and my confidence in their final triumph. Chang looked up with an unexpectedly grim expression. His voice had a bitterness that had not been there before.

'You think we've done pretty well do you? I can tell you that we've only taken the first step in our 10,000 li Long March. All the figures I've given you are true but the important thing, the really decisive thing, has been the class struggle. We've had to fight every inch of the way against those who would turn us back. In future we'll still have to fight. If we drop our guard, relax our vigilance, we'll be beaten. We'll lose all that we've gained. That's the important thing to understand. We can only beat schistosomiasis so long as we keep on the socialist road. If we turn off that road, the snails will win and we shall lose.'

His tension passed. 'If I were you, I'd spend a day or two in Ren Tun village in the south-west of this county. That village used to have more than its share of schistosomiasis. If you talk with the villagers there, you will see this disease in human, not just in statistical terms'.

I decided to go to Ren Tun.

THE VILLAGE THAT CAME TO LIFE

The only way to get to Ren Tun is by boat. The boatman nosed his way through a maze of channels with skill and certainty. Once we skirted the fringe of a lake so vast that we couldn't see its distant shore but we soon left it for narrow waterways flanked by cultivated fields of every tint of green, hidden now and then by riverside bamboo groves undulating in the breeze like silken gowns. We met other boatmen, some in stately sailing craft laden with bags of grain or cement, some in rowing boats casting circular fishing nets on the waters like cowboys demonstrating their skill with lassoes, some straining at huge single oars as they towed cavalcades of bamboo logs through the green waters.

Soon I heard a faint boom of drums and as we turned a corner, I could see a group of villagers with red flags and brass instruments glinting in the sunshine. We had arrived.

They waved and shouted as our boat slid alongside. A scarlet streamer spanned the river, yellow characters spelling out a welcome to 'international friend Hung Ro Shi' (my Chinese name). Cymbals clashed with redoubled enthusiasm as a boy and a girl helped me ashore and led me to a guard of honour of Young Pioneers, rosy cheeked, white shirted, red scarved. Their representative stepped forward, saluted smartly, tied a scarf around my neck and made a formal little speech of welcome. The children clapped and waved and pressed round me. The grown-ups looked on, laughing, making a huge noise with their percussion instruments, full of warmth and welcome.

I would like to have said a few words in reply but none would come.

We sat on trestles in a lofty room with a beaten earth floor. The glassless windows overlooked the river and a succession of grubby-faced children peered in to get a glimpse of the strange visitor. Sometimes one would sneak into the room, willing himself into the shadows, and sit cross-legged on the floor. All too soon he would be discovered and shooed out.

One after another the peasants told me about themselves and their village.

First Comrade Wu Hai Qan, vice-director of the Ren Tun production brigade, regaled me with facts and figures.

'In this village we have 1,327 mu of cultivated land and 183 families totalling 671 people organized in five production teams. In the old days, in addition to the burdens which weighed us all down, we had the burden of schistosomiasis. It pressed us sorely and all but wiped us out. In the twenty years from 1930 to 1949, 500 died in this village. The living hardly had the strength to bury the dead. Ninety-seven families died out completely and twenty families had only one survivor each. By the time of Liberation only 461 people were left of whom 449 had schistosomiasis. We didn't know anything about the disease, not even its name. We just called it big belly disease. Some thought it wasn't a disease at all but a punishment for some sin committed by our ancestors.

'I knew a poor peasant called Ren Chang. We used to play together as children. He grew up and married and there were five in his family. Then his father and mother died of big belly disease and he went to work for the landlord. One day he vomited blood and the landlord sent him home without a penny piece for eight months work. He knew there was no hope for him so he strangled himself. Soon after, his wife and children died and the whole family was wiped out.

'Our Party secretary had fifteen in his family; he is the only survivor. In the second production team there is a family called Lu. Of the forty-five in his family, thirty died within a few years. All you could see in his house were ancestral tablets.

'The survivors were so weak that they could hardly grow enough grain for their needs. No child was born here for seven years before Liberation. We forgot the music of a baby's laughter. People used to write verses about our village.

> "Ren Tun folk all grow on vines
> Faces yellow like old pumpkins
> Scrawny limbs like unripe gourds,
> Swollen bellies, water filled
> Tight and smooth as water-melons."

"This dread disease has brought disaster to our village.

Death stalks the land and puts a ban on birth.
Our daughters long to leave and marry into healthier climes."

"Eastern neighbour, prematurely old,
    Mourns for the young ones, dead before their time.
Western neighbour, still a child
    Weeps for his still unburied parents." '

As Comrade Wu reminisced and recited the sad poems of yesteryear, others joined in and the atmosphere became more and more gloomy. Suddenly he changed the subject. 'Enough of that stuff,' he said. 'That's no way to treat a guest. Let's tell him of the changes in our village. You tell him, old Guan, you were Party secretary even before Liberation when the Party was still underground. You know more about it than anyone else.'

Old Guan, nearly toothless, with deeply wrinkled dark brown face and shaven head, produced a sheaf of notes. 'To put it briefly, there have been four big changes here since Liberation.

'Firstly, the population has risen from 461 to 671. Sixty-seven of our men have married, many of them bringing brides from other villages.

'Secondly, rice production has gone up from 400 to 786 jin[1] per mu and there are now 859 pigs in the village as compared with none in 1949.

'Thirdly, income has gone up from an average of forty yuan per able-bodied worker per year to 137 yuan. More than 150 houses have been built and many more have been renovated.

'Fourthly, all our children now go to school, whereas formerly there were only five literates in the village and three of them were from landlord families. We have two primary schools of our own and nearly twenty children attend middle school in a neighbouring village.

'As for health, there is simply no comparison. It's true that we still have some cases of schistosomiasis but there are hardly any new ones and we haven't found any live snails for months. Seven of our youths have been accepted by the People's Liberation Army and everyone knows how high their physical requirements are. We have two basket-ball teams and last year we were the county champions. Just imagine! Ren Tun folk running about for the fun of it! In the old days we could hardly run if there was a tiger on our heels.' He turned to me with a twinkle in his eye. 'Would you like to see our basket-ball teams practising?'

I said that I would, but another peasant broke in, and started to tell me about himself.

'I had four brothers and sisters and three of them died of big belly disease before I was eight years old. Then my mother died and only my father, my elder brother and I were left. My father was the strongest man in the village. But he was superstitious and when my brother started to get thin and yellow, my father told him to go round all the temples to collect magic incense ash. But he got worse and worse. My father heard of a famous folk doctor who could cure this disease if he was paid enough money. So we sold our land and my father took my brother to the doctor, taking me too because I was too little

[1] 1 jin = 1·1 pounds.

to be left. I'll always remember that doctor. He had the longest white beard I've ever seen and he was the cruellest man in the world. He felt my brother's spleen and said it had grown eyes and he'd have to blind them. So he took a metal spike, made it red hot and stuck it into my brother's belly. My brother screamed and fainted but the doctor said it was all right because he had blinded the spleen and we could go home now.

'We went home, my father carrying my brother all the way. The wound in his belly went septic and soon after that my brother died.

'A few months later, my father got sick and although he was so strong, he died within the year.

'I was all alone and very frightened. I ran away to another village and lived in a temple where there was a clay god named Wang. I changed my surname to his and prayed to him to take me as his foster-son. I swore that if he did, I would keep him in good repair and look after all his needs. I got a job with a landlord who beat me, drove me and starved me. Liberation came just in time or my bones would long since have rotted.'

One of the few women present broke the momentary silence.

'I married when I was twenty-four years of age and when my belly started to swell, I thought I was pregnant. But it was the God of Plague who had lodged in my belly. After Liberation I got some injections which made me feel very bad. But my disease gradually got better and when I was forty-four my belly started to swell again. This time it was a real pregnancy. I had a lovely little daughter and on her first birthday I had her photo taken and sent it to Chairman Mao. He sent me a nice letter back.'

Old Wu looked at the darkening sky. 'If we don't watch the basket-ball now it will be too late.' We filed out and walked to the basket-ball pitch where the game was already in progress. They were certainly very good, strong and quick with excellent team work. A toothless old granny who, in her old age, had become a basket-ball fan, cackled appreciatively. 'That one over there is my grandson, Just think of it! Playing ball for fun! In the old days most of us Ren Tun folk had a big ball in our bellies—not in our hands. What a change in our lives. I still don't properly understand what's happened.'

The sun was sinking as we strolled back. My hosts urged me to have supper with them so that we could continue to talk for as long as we liked. 'Just ordinary food. Our own produce.' It was their own produce but it was far from ordinary. We had fish and prawns from the lake, vegetables of all kinds, broad beans, wild mushrooms, duck eggs, water-chestnuts and fragrant fresh-husked rice. Food was piled on my plate and I was urged to eat and to eat until I stood up and said it was getting late and I wanted to hear more.

We went back to the big room, now lit by a hurricane lamp, and talked of the past, the present and the future. Unexpectedly, a swarthy, freckled, broad-shouldered young woman with bobbed hair started talking. 'My name is Lu Zhing Zhuan. I'd like to tell you about my father. I haven't spoken of it since it happened but it was so long ago that now I can tell the story without pain. I think it should be told.

'My family was very poor. We were fisher-folk and lived on our boat. Mother died when we children were very young and father brought us up. He was a bitter man and seldom smiled or played with us. But he worked from dawn to dusk and did whatever he could for us. Then his belly started to swell and he got so thin and weak that he could hardly row the boat. There was a doctor in the county town who could draw off fluid from the belly. My father borrowed money and went to the doctor who drew off the fluid. After that my father was much better but soon his belly swelled again and he could borrow no more money. His brother lived on the boat with us and he too had big belly disease. One night he fell overboard and was drowned. The neighbours said he didn't fall but jumped.

'My father couldn't work and I did the fishing myself. But I couldn't pull in the nets properly and one day I tore them and the shrimps all escaped. My father was very angry and beat me. He was really angry with himself because he couldn't work and as he beat me he cried and the more he cried the more he beat me.

'He got weaker and weaker and could hardly stand. Then he told me to get an awl and a duck quill and make a hole in his belly and put the duck quill in it to draw off the water. I refused and he beat me again. I was so sorry for him that I got the duck quill and borrowed an awl used for sewing cloth shoes. He showed me where to make the hole but I just couldn't do it.

'I clutched his legs but he beat me, sobbing as he did so, and pleaded with me to do it. So I did. It was quite easy. I stuck the awl in just below the belly button. His belly was as tight as a drum and as I pulled the awl out, I pushed the quill in. Water squirted out of the duck quill. I got a bucket and before long it was nearly full. I was staggered. My father lay on his side with water squirting out of the quill. A neighbour came over from the next boat and emptied the bucket. He brought us some food but nobody could eat it.

'Next day my father was very ill. He told me to go to the temples for magic pills and to tell the priests that he would rebuild the temples when he got better. He died in three days. Before he died he looked so terrible, so thin and yellow and his lips and tongue were black. I'll never forget it. I didn't even know when he died. He just became still and stopped groaning. A neighbour came and said he was dead. We had no money to bury him so we wrapped him in an old sail and put him into the water.

'My brother became a cowherd and I became a child labourer in a factory.'

She talked in a torrent, so fast that I could hardly write down what she said. I asked her to speak more slowly but she poured out a flood of words as though she was expelling the accumulated bitterness of a lifetime. Her face was torn with emotion but she was dry-eyed.

I tried to console her, to tell her that she should feel no remorse since her father would have died anyway. 'Remorse! I feel no remorse. We were both victims of the old society—both my father and I and so were many thousands of others.' She was shouting now—her face suffused with anger. 'I hate the old society. I hate it. And I will smash the skull of anyone who tries to bring it back again!'

Then the tears came. But they were tears of anger, not of grief; tears of relief for the ending of the nightmare of the past.

11
Scaling the peaks

In May 1942, when the Japanese Imperial Army had occupied the greater part of China, when Chiang Kai-shek had withdrawn to his mountain stronghold in the South-West to conserve his strength for dealing with the 'Red Peril', when part of the Communist army, possessing only millet and rifles, was blockaded in the barren hills of the North-West, a month long conference on Literature and Art was held in Yenan, the Communist capital.

It may seem strange that under such stringent conditions, so much time could be devoted to an apparently academic discussion. Actually it was not strange. Men unite and fight to the extent that they know what they are fighting for and love what they know. Stories, books, songs and plays are munitions of war just as much as bombs and bullets.

Chairman Mao made two memorable speeches at this conference, speeches which continue to guide not only literary and art workers but also other professional workers such as doctors.

Their main theme is that the over-riding and abiding duty of professional workers is to serve the interests of the mass of the people and in the course of doing so, progressively to refine and upgrade their work.

Most of this book describes how medicine in China serves the labouring people. This chapter describes three fields of endeavour in which Chinese medical scientists have scaled the peaks of science.

BURNS
During the momentous year of 1958, when the Chinese people 'stormed the heavens', the importance of steel production in the national economy became clear to everybody and home-made steel converters sprouted like mushrooms.

My son, then a fourteen-year-old schoolboy, didn't come home for forty-eight hours and then he turned up, grimy, dishevelled, exhausted but triumphant. 'We made it, Dad,' he announced excitedly. 'We turned out our first heat of steel. The quality is not very good yet. It's not up to standard. But the next lot, or the one after that, will be.'

Many people have sneered at China's steel campaign as 'wasteful', 'a big flop', 'fanaticism', etc. In my opinion, and in the opinion of many others, the steel campaign, while it involved a certain amount of waste, had positive aspects that greatly outweighed the negative. It spread knowledge of steel smelting throughout the land and laid the foundations for self-sufficiency.

On the last day of May, 1958, a Shanghai steel worker named Chiu Tsai Kang was splashed by molten steel. His clothes caught fire and he sustained burns covering eighty-nine per cent of the entire surface of the body.

He was rushed to the Kwangtzu Hospital, Shanghai, where a drama began to unfold which was to have repercussions lasting to the present day and extending far beyond the borders of China.

According to scientifically worked out statistics from the most advanced centres for the treatment of burns in Britain and USA, his chances of survival

107

were almost nil. The question was whether, at a time when China was crashing through centuries, the Chinese people should accept the experience of other countries as setting a limit for what they could or could not accomplish; whether People's China, for all its technical backwardness, could provide better treatment for a burned worker than Western countries could provide for monarchs and millionaires. A burn of such magnitude,was a challenge and the times demanded that the challenge be met.

In the early stages, shock due to loss of fluid from the burned area was the main danger. As soon as the public learnt that blood and plasma were needed in large quantities, a constant stream of volunteer blood donors presented themselves at the hospital. In the first twenty-three days of treatment, he received 30,700 ccs of blood and plasma, about six times the total volume of blood in his body.

If he survived the shock phase, infection would become the main danger, for a burn is, in effect, a huge open wound and severe infection can easily lead to septicaemia and death.

Within twenty-four hours a special air-conditioned suite of rooms was set up exclusively for the treatment of this one patient. Filtered, humidified and temperature controlled air was blown in under positive pressure and evacuated to the exterior through special vents. All personnel entering the treatment block were required to bathe and change into sterile clothing. Nurses volunteered to cut off their plaits in the interests of hygiene.

The Party Committee in the hospital called a number of conferences attended by doctors, nurses and representatives of ordinary hospital workers such as cooks, cleaners, maintenance workers and boilermen, to work out short-term and long-term plans.

Four doctors, eight nurses and a team of laboratory workers, orderlies and cooks were allocated to care for the patient on a round-the-clock basis.

Experts in related fields such as bacteriology, pharmacology, biochemistry, plastic surgery, haematology and immunology were flown into Shanghai from all over China. I was among them and, like most of the others, I learned more than I taught, received more than I gave.

At a time when he most needed nourishment, the patient's appetite started to flag. Protein-rich fluid was continuously being discharged from the huge wound, and he wasted visibly. The hospital dietician tempted him with every dish he could think of, but day by day he ate less and less. When news of this leaked out, the chefs of Shanghai's famous restaurants put their heads together. They produced specimen menus, different ones for every meal, and sent a stream of delicacies to the hospital. His comrades urged him to eat as a political duty, as his contribution to the fight for his life that was being waged with such determination by so many. Chiu responded to the best of his ability.

Then the dead skin sloughed away, leaving a huge raw area with bones and joints exposed where the burn had been deepest. The only way to heal such a wound is by skin-grafting which involves cutting very thin sheets of skin from the unburned areas and applying them to the raw surface. The sheets of skin are cut so thin that the donor areas from which they are cut heal by themselves within two or three weeks. However, in a burn as big as this one, the unburnt areas from which grafts can be cut are so small that one is forced to apply grafts sparingly only to those parts which need it most and wait for the donor areas to heal so that a second or a third lot of skin grafts can be cut from the same place. This delays complete grafting and time is a very important factor in the treatment of burns for the longer the wound remains unhealed, the greater the loss of protein, the more prolonged the fever, the more debilitating the infection and the greater the risk of complications. The treatment of a really extensive burn is a race against time. Everything that speeds up healing increases the chance of survival; everything that delays it, increases the danger.

It would be ideal if skin from another donor could be used to heal the burn but although a great deal of research work has been done, up to the present time only the patient's own skin can effect a permanent cure. Homografts, that is skin grafts from another donor, usually 'take' in the same way as the patient's own skin but after a few weeks they gradually melt away and disappear. This is because the body develops an immunological reaction to the 'foreign skin' in the same way as it does to germs.

However, although skin homografts do not take permanently, they can be life-saving in the treatment of very big burns since until they disappear, they effectively heal the burn and during this time the general condition improves dramatically. The temperature comes down, the appetite and the nutrition improve, the anaemia gets less, pain is alleviated and the patient's own donor areas heal up and can yield further skin grafts.

For these reasons, skin from healthy persons was extensively used in the treatment of Chiu Tsai Kang. Hundreds of would-be skin donors came to the hospital, telephoned, wrote letters, begging to be allowed to donate skin. The senior surgeon in the hospital was one of the first to volunteer.

Every day a whole series of bacteriological, haematological and biochemical tests were carried out which, in the whole course of treatment, must have run into thousands.

Interest in his progress was nation-wide. Daily bulletins were issued and it became necessary for the hospital to open a special office to deal with inquiries.

Eventually the wounds were all healed and his life was saved. This was a great victory which not only rejoiced people everywhere, but also provided an impetus to the treatment of burns which makes itself felt to this day.

Hundreds of doctors had been directly or indirectly involved in the treatment of Chiu Tsai Kang. When they returned home and reported back, hospitals throughout the country made arrangements for the treatment of severe burns. In my own hospital we opened a special burns ward, trained nursing and medical staff, and embarked on a research programme to answer some outstanding questions.

Our first patient died. His total area of burning was slightly less than that of Chiu Tsai Kang, but the area of deep burning was greater, amounting to seventy per cent of the body area. In order to turn the patient painlessly, without touching him, we needed a special turning bed.

Our hospital maintenance workers made it for us within twelve hours.

By the twelfth day the burnt skin started to separate and his condition deteriorated. We held an emergency consultation and it was suggested that

109

to help drainage from the burn he should lie on an air mattress which could be inflated or deflated in sections. No such mattresses existed. It was nearly midnight and the patient was desperately ill. A colleague and I went to a tiny back-street factory which made plastic raincoats and we explained our idea to the few workers who were on night shift. They summoned the day shift workers, with them drew a sketch of the proposed mattress, modified it according to suggestions and, as dawn was breaking, produced a twelve-section plastic air mattress, each section independently inflatable and deflatable. None of the men had ever seen or heard of such a mattress before.

Three days later the patient died of septicaemia. Just after he died, a worker from the raincoat factory telephoned to say that they had made a better air mattress. We told him the sad news and he said that if we planned to hold a memorial meeting, he and his mates would like to attend as they felt that they had taken part in his treatment.

Hospitals throughout the country rapidly gained experience in the treatment of extensive burns. Teams of experienced doctors and nurses were flown out on request, a great deal of research work was undertaken and many national and provincial conferences were held.

Reports appeared in the Chinese medical press of bigger and bigger burns being successfully treated. I recently saw a successful case where the only unburnt skin was on the sole of one foot, the toes of both feet and the crown of the head. From these areas crop after crop of tiny skin grafts were harvested until the enormous burn was healed.

As experience was gained, mortality and the duration of hospitalization fell.

By 1964 sufficient material had been accumulated to enable us to compare our results with those reported by leading Burns Centres in other countries and we were pleased to discover that within six years we had caught up with or even surpassed them.

For example, Dr T. G. Blocker,[1] an American expert, analyzed the mortality in a thousand cases of burns. His findings and comparable figures for the Kwang Tzu Hospital in Shanghai are as follows:

Area of Burn (Percentage of body area)	Mortality Rate	
	Blocker, USA	Shanghai Kwangtzu Hospital
51-60%	54·9%	33·3%
61-70%	77·2%	43·3%
over 71%	94·7%	67·9%

Although China has reached a high level in the treatment of burns, we certainly cannot be satisfied with these results and many problems still have to be solved.

The most serious problem is that achieving these results demands an enormous expenditure of manpower and resources. We have not yet found a way to simplify treatment so as to bring it within the reach of every hospital and clinic.

Another problem is that, although we can now save the lives of patients with

[1] Blocker. *Journal of Traumatology*. 1. 409. 1961.

enormous burns, many of the survivors are severely handicapped and disfigured. Chiu Tsai Kang, for example, is now back at work in the steel mill where he sustained his burns, but his joints were so stiff after he recovered from the burn that it took a year's physiotherapy before he was able to walk. The first time he put on his shirt it took him more than an hour since he couldn't put his arm behind his back.

We now direct our efforts towards the preservation of function in addition to the saving of life. We are confident that in time we shall solve these and other problems, for the prevailing atmosphere in China is one of determination to surmount all difficulties in the service of the people, of confidence, of respect for science and of nation-wide co-operation which ensures that every advance is put at the disposal of all who can benefit from it.

TOTAL SYNTHESIS OF BIOLOGICALLY ACTIVE BOVINE INSULIN

Ninety years ago, Frederick Engels, co-founder with Karl Marx of the theory of scientific socialism, wrote: 'Life is the mode of existence of protein bodies . . . as soon as the composition of protein bodies becomes known, chemistry will be able to set about the preparation of living protein.'

It is no accident that the world's first total synthesis of a biologically active protein was carried out in socialist China, by scientists armed with the theory of Marx and Engels, now immeasurably deepened and enriched by Mao Tse-tung, thereby strikingly confirming Engels' brilliant insight.

Engels was concerned about protein science because it impinged on a question intimately connected with the essence of the controversy between philosophical materialists and philosophical idealists, the question of the origin of life. Marx and Engels were materialists maintaining that life has resulted from the movement, evolution and development of inorganic matter over millions of years. Idealists, on the contrary, believe that life is essentially unknowable and mysterious, created by God or by a supernatural force and that the gulf between living and non-living matter is unbridgeable and absolute. They used to maintain that a similar gap existed between organic and inorganic substances but when the German scientist Wöhler synthesized the organic compound urea from inorganic substances in 1828, he showed that the gulf was not insurmountable.

What is insulin?

Insulin is the simplest of all proteins. It is a hormone produced by groups of cells in the pancreas of man and other mammals, which has the important function of helping the combustion in the body of sugar, the end-product of carbohydrates, the main energy-giving foods. Failure of the pancreas to produce insulin is the cause of diabetes, a disease in which sugar cannot be fully utilized by the tissues so that its level in the blood rises until it overflows into the urine.

The physiochemical structure of insulin was worked out by Sanger and his colleagues in Cambridge after nearly ten years of intensive research work which was rewarded with the Nobel Prize. It was found to consist of two chains of peptides, the A chain containing twenty-one amino acids and the B chain containing thirty amino acids linked together by two disulphide

111

linkages, one between the seventh amino acid in the A chain and the seventh in the B chain, and another between the twentieth in the A chain and the nineteenth in the B chain. In addition, there is a disulphide linkage between the sixth and eleventh amino acids in the A chain.

The structure of insulin is shown diagrammatically below:—

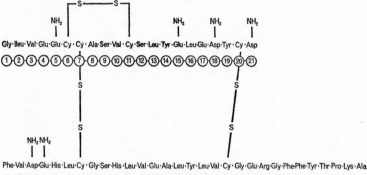

The structure of insulin.

However, even though insulin is the simplest protein, it is still very complex, for the description and the diagram refer only to its primary structure. The two peptide chains are in fact not straight but are coiled into helical shapes which give the molecule its secondary structure and the coiled chains are again folded in space in a distinctive pattern which constitutes its tertiary structure. This coiling and folding is not haphazard but very precise and specific, and confers on the protein its biological activity.

As soon as the structure of the molecule was known, the task of synthesizing it appeared on the agenda of scientists all over the world. The difficulties, however, were so formidable that the British magazine *Nature* carried an editorial which stated that 'the possibility that insulin may be synthesized in the laboratory . . . is unlikely to occur for some time to come.'

That editorial was published in 1958. In the same year the Chinese Communist Party put out its General Line calling on the people to go all out and aim high. In the same year the Great Leap Forward got under way. In the same year a small group of young biochemists in Shanghai decided to synthesize insulin.

Why insulin?

When I asked these young scientists why they decided to synthesize insulin, a lively discussion followed and it became clear that there was not one reason but many and that they did not all carry equal weight with each member of the team.

It was a response to the call of the Party to go all out and aim high, a response to the spirit of the Great Leap.

It was a challenge. Could China, which until Liberation couldn't even make a motor-car, let alone synthesize protein, compete with famous scientists from the technically advanced countries in pursuit of this elusive goal?

It would strike a blow at idealism and strengthen the dialectical materialist conception of the universe which was increasingly becoming the world outlook and guide to action of millions of Chinese.

It would open up new fields in science, would start to lift the curtain of ignorance concerning the origin of life.

It would make possible the synthesis of human insulin which is chemically not quite identical with bovine insulin, and this might be of value in the treatment of certain rare cases of diabetes.

It might even, one day, lead to the possibility of the large-scale synthesis of protein for human consumption and make a contribution to the feeding of the human race.

It was a rebellion against domination by established authorities who habitually poured cold water on the enthusiasm of the young, urged circumspection, told them not to try to run before they could walk, emphasized the difficulties and cautioned them against aiming too high. The Chinese educational system had its roots in the old society where the professor usually decided on major research topics and the juniors carried them out. The professor, either foreign trained or servile to foreign science, would usually select a research project from those reported in foreign journals, being content to follow in the footsteps of Western scientists, keeping a respectful distance behind them, never doing anything really original, never contradicting them and certainly not daring to compete with them.

In the heady gusts of the Great Leap, the young scientists in the Shanghai Institute of Biochemistry rebelled against their fusty old professors with their reverence for everything foreign and their distrust of everything Chinese, and decided to synthesize insulin. They were not anti-authority or anti-foreign. They were against the trammels which prevented them from giving expression to their desire to respond to the spirit of the times, to the call of Chairman Mao and to do something in their own field that would bring credit to their country.

Strategy and tactics

Theoretically, there were many different ways of going about the synthesis of insulin.

If the insulin molecule could be split in half transversely, across the two chains, and the two halves joined up again, a molecule would result which, with suitable modifications, might be changed into insulin.

Alternatively, it might be possible to synthesize insulin by elongating the peptide cystine, adding amino acid groupings in the correct sequence until something resembling insulin resulted.

Alternatively, those parts of the molecule containing the disulphide linkages could be synthesized separately and then joined together.

But the most promising approach was that of synthesizing the A and B chains separately and then joining them together with disulphide linkages in the correct places. This method has the great advantage that it could be done in two stages. The first stage would be to split natural insulin into its A and B chains and then try to join the chains together to reconstitute active insulin. If this succeeded, the next stage would be to make synthetic chains and then join them together. If it failed, they would be unlikely to succeed in joining synthetic chains and another approach must be sought before embarking on the immensely laborious task of synthesizing the A and B chains.

This method was therefore chosen as the basic strategy. The disposition of forces then had to be worked out. The main force was the group of biochemists in the Institute of Biochemistry, but since the work would involve disciplines other than biochemistry, the Department of Chemistry at Peking University and the Institute of Organic Chemistry were invited to co-operate. They agreed to do so and formed teams which worked closely together for the next six and a half years.

In addition to these three main groups, fifteen other small groups were established for co-operation on particular aspects of the project.

At the outset, the average age of the scientists involved was twenty-five years.

Overcoming difficulties

One of the early obstacles was the negative attitude of some of the established authorities to the whole project. Lacking confidence themselves, they tried to undermine the confidence of the young scientists, deriding them as 'loafers in fur coats' and sneering at the project as an 'idiot's day-dream'. This kind of attack became particularly vicious during the three hard years 1959-61 when the General Line and the Great Leap came under fire.

Since these attacks were essentially political in nature, the young scientists countered them by strengthening their own political standpoint, studying the works of Chairman Mao, mingling with workers and peasants and learning from them courage and resolution in the face of difficulties. Leading members of the Central Committee of the Party encouraged them, saying that even if they didn't succeed, their descendants would carry on from where they left off and would certainly achieve success.

Another difficulty was their lack of experience. They learned as they went along and turned their mistakes into successes by drawing lessons from them.

'If a man wants to succeed in his work . . . he must bring his ideas into correspondence with the laws of the objective external world; if they do not correspond, he will fail in his practice. After he fails, he draws his lessons, corrects his ideas . . . and can thus turn failure into success; this is what is meant by "failure is the mother of Success" and "a fall into the pit, a gain in your wit".[1]

In this way, in the course of practical work, they gradually overcame the problem of inexperience.

Another difficulty was their lack of equipment. They had no apparatus for the identification of polypeptides, China completely lacked a fine chemical reagent industry, only a few amino acids were available in China and to import them in the quantities needed would be very expensive. One of the amino acids in insulin costs 120 yuan (£20) a gram.

[1] Mao Tse-tung 'On Practice'. July 1937. *Selected Works, Vol. I, pp.* 296-7.

Scientists, technicians and workers in the chemical industry joined forces and before long had established a completely new branch of industry which largely solved the problem of fine chemical reagents. At the same time they made the necessary apparatus for the identification and separation of amino acids and within six months, all seventeen amino acids in insulin had been made in sufficient quantities to enable the work to proceed.

Still another problem concerned the secondary and tertiary structure of insulin. Even if they could synthesize the long A and B chains and join them up so as to reproduce the primary structure of insulin, what guarantee was there that they could reproduce the secondary and tertiary structure, the coiling and folding of the chains in space?

To answer this basic question was one of the main objectives of the early stages of the project. There were two viewpoints. One was that the secondary and tertiary structure of protein molecules was determined by mysterious factors beyond the control or understanding of man. The other was that, if the necessary conditions could be discovered and created, the primary structure itself would determine the secondary and tertiary structures.

Milestones on the way

The first stage of the work was to split natural insulin into its A and B chains and then join them up in the right way.

For thirty years, scientists in many countries had been trying to cleave the insulin molecule into two parts and reconstitute them into biologically active insulin. The Chinese scientists succeeded in this task after one year's work and reported it in January 1960. In the same year Dixon and Wardlaw also succeeded in reconstituting insulin from its separated A and B chains but the activity of their product was from 1-2% and it could not be purified or crystallized, whereas the Chinese workers obtained first a 5-10% activity then 50% activity and finally 100% activity from a purified, crystallized product.

The first hurdle had been crossed. The conditions under which natural A and B chains could be rejoined were now understood and it was known that mastery of these conditions also gave mastery over the spatial arrangements which determined the higher ordered structure and biological activity of insulin.

While this work was going on, other scientists were busy synthesizing and extracting the necessary amino acids. Then came the exceedingly laborious task of joining up the synthesized amino acids in the right sequence and with the right linkages. Both A and B chains were longer than any peptide chains which had ever been synthesized and the addition of each amino acid caused some loss of what had already been accomplished so that the amount of pure material became progressively less as the chains became longer.

By 1964, both A and B chains had been synthesized and the text task was to make a 'hybrid' molecule, one half of which was natural and the other half synthetic. First a synthetic B chain was joined to a natural A chain and then a synthetic A chain to a natural B chain. This could be called semi-synthesis and the resultant hybrid insulin in each case showed from 5-10% activity.

115

Towards the end of 1964, they succeeded in joining synthetic A and B chains together but the biological activity of the product was so low that it was impossible to extract pure crystallized insulin from it. The whole process of synthesizing the A and B chains was reviewed and modified in order to secure a more stable and purer product at every stage.

Eventually a crude substance with from 1·2% to 2·5% of the activity of natural insulin was produced and after repeated extraction with an acidified secondary butanol solvent system, its activity increased more than tenfold.

On 17 September, 1965, cubical crystals resembling those of transparent quartz were obtained and were later proved to be crystals of pure bovine insulin. Total synthesis of a complete, biologically active protein had been accomplished for the first time in history.

Proof

It remained only to prove that the crystalline substance which was the fruit of six and a half years of intensive work, was in fact insulin, and such proof was not difficult to obtain.

The size, shape, solubility and other characteristics of the crystals were identical with those of natural insulin.

Its biological properties when tested in a variety of ways were also identical. For example, insulin causes convulsions when injected into a mouse and a comparison of the amounts of natural and synthetic insulin needed to cause convulsions showed that natural insulin contains 23·7 International Units per milligram, and synthetic insulin, 24.

The natural and the synthetic substances had identical effects in lowering the blood sugar of a rabbit.

The results of chemical testing by electro-phoresis showed an identity between the natural and synthetic substances.

The two substances gave the same 'fingerprints' after enzymic digestion and chromatography.

An anti-insulin serum produced by natural insulin completely neutralized the synthetic substance and vice versa.

As final proof, a batch of unpurified synthetic insulin was made in which the glycine amino acid group in the A chain had been labelled with a radioactive carbon isotope. It was then mixed with natural insulin and purified in stages. The ratio of radioactivity to biological activity remained constant at all stages of purification showing a complete identity between the natural and synthetic substance.

Who did it?

It was getting late when the group of young scientists had succeeded in giving me an elementary understanding of their work. I was really out of my depth and they had used up several blackboards in an attempt to reduce the subject to a simplicity which even I could grasp.

When I congratulated them on their tremendous achievement they brushed that aside. 'Our achievements are all in the past,' they said. 'What matters is what we do in the future. If we dwell in the past we shall become conceited and backward. There is nothing for us to be conceited about. When we were

116

guided by the thinking of Chairman Mao, we made progress; when we were not, we went astray.

'For example, the B chain is very insoluble and at first we saw this as a stumbling block and were dispirited. But Chairman Mao teaches us that bad things can become good things and so we utilized the insolubility of the B chain as a method of separation and purification.

'Whenever we were confronted by a problem and couldn't see the way forward we tried to find out what was the principal contradiction, for Mao says: "There are many contradictions in the process of development of a complex thing and one of them is necessarily the principal contradiction whose existence and development determines or influences the existence or development of the other contradictions."[1] At one stage, when we seemed to be at an impasse, we analyzed the principal contradiction as being between the necessity to reproduce the higher ordered structure of the insulin molecule and our inability to do so. So we concentrated exclusively on this problem and once we had mastered the conditions for combining natural A and B chains in the right way, we were able to forge ahead.'

I asked who had been chiefly responsible for the work but they would mention no names at all. 'It's been a collective job from start to finish and we don't intend to single out any individuals. The division of labour has been according to the needs of the project. Any of us could have done any part of it.'

I left the laboratory with the feeling that China's new generation of audacious young scientists will storm many more citadels and ensure a leading position for China in the world of science.

REATTACHMENT OF SEVERED LIMBS

On 2 January 1963, a young man named Wang Cung Po severed his right hand above the wrist when he caught it in a machine. An ambulance was called and within minutes he was on his way to the Sixth Municipal Hospital, Shanghai. His workmate, an old factory worker, looked under Wang's lathe and found the severed hand still in its protective glove. He picked it up, noted that it was still warm and decided to take it to the hospital. 'You'd better wrap it up,' he was told, 'or the passengers on the bus will be scared stiff.' So he got a clean towel from the toilet and arrived at the hospital just as Dr Chen, the surgeon on duty, was discussing the case with his junior colleagues. It wasn't very complicated. The hand had been cut off and that was that. It would be easy enough to shorten the bones and stitch the skin flaps together over the end of the stump so that later on he could be fitted with an artificial hand.

It would be easy enough and yet Dr Chen didn't feel at all happy about it. He had recently spent some weeks working in a factory and had acquired a great respect for the industriousness and character of factory workers. An artificial hand looked like a real one but workers were concerned with reality, not with appearances. And the reality was that a one-handed worker was practically useless.

The veteran worker knocked at the door, came in, unwrapped the severed hand and laid it on the desk. 'Seems a pity not to use it,' he said. 'It's still

[1] 'On Contradiction' Mao Tse-tung. *Selected Works, Vol.* 1, *p.* 331.

warm and there isn't a mark on it. I know you surgeons are doing wonderful things nowadays, putting artificial valves into hearts and such like. Do you think you could put it back on again?'

The operation took seven hours.

The blood clots in the blood vessels of the severed hand were washed out with a substance which could prevent further clotting. All bruised and damaged tissues were carefully removed to prevent infection and the bones were securely joined together with stainless steel plates, screws and wires. When the crucial step of joining up the arteries had been completed and blood was allowed to flow through them, the waxen hand flushed pink and its veins became distended. Two veins were then joined up and the cut nerves and tendons were repaired using a special technique to prevent adhesions.

After the operation, doctors and nurses kept a round-the-clock vigil. They took hourly temperature readings from the fingertips of the reattached hand with an electric skin thermometer and found that the temperature was actually higher than on the normal side.

On the second day, disaster threatened. The hand started to swell and to cool down. A consultation was called and all agreed that unless some means could be found to stop the swelling, the hand was doomed. One surgeon who had carried out experiments in reattaching dogs' legs, had found that once a reattached limb started to swell, the only way to save it was to make incisions into it so that the fluid could drain out. That is what was done to Wang Cung Po's hand, and in the course of the next few days the swelling gradually subsided and the hand again became warm and pink.

The following year at a Surgical Congress in Peking, surgeons from all over the world reported on their country's outstanding achievements. For me, the highlight of the congress was a speech made by the young worker, Wang Cung Po, who mounted the rostrum dressed in his blue denims and, without a trace of shyness, told the distinguished guests about his reattached hand. 'My father used to work in a factory,' he said. 'One day a machine fell on his foot and smashed it. He was driven out without a penny of compensation and never managed to find another job because he walked with a limp. My right hand was cut off but the doctors put it back on again and trained me to use it. My factory waited patiently for me to recover the use of my hand and they paid me my full wages all the time.'

'Here is the hand,' he said as with a dramatic and intensely moving gesture he raised his right arm and clenched and unclenched the fist. 'My right hand has been given back to me by our socialist society. I swear that I will use it till my dying day to safeguard our good new life.'

Some three years later, on a visit to Shanghai, I got in touch with Wang Cung Po. He was working at his original job, had become a skilled inventor, was deeply immersed in the Cultural Revolution and was a leading member of the Rebel Group in his factory. 'You remember,' he said, 'that I swore to safeguard our socialist society. That's why I joined the Rebel Group, for we're rebelling against those who would prefer our country to become capitalist. That's why I give every minute of my free time to the Cultural Revolution because its purpose is to make sure that China stays red for ever.'

Using plastic tubing, he had made me a model of a prawn of such artistry

118

and perfection of craftsmanship that the function in the reattached hand must have been excellent. His hand was completely normal in colour, temperature, and texture. Movements of the fingers were practically full but wrist movements were slightly limited and careful testing showed that the skin was not quite as sensitive as the skin on the other hand. He uses the hand normally, does gymnastics and is a keen ping-pong player.

The long-term result in this first case of reattachment of a completely severed hand is extraordinarily good.

The exceptional becomes the commonplace

The successful reattachment of a completely severed limb is undoubtedly a triumph of surgery but if only one patient benefits from this triumph, then it cannot have much social significance. The next task therefore was to popularize this advance, to place it at the service of all people with limbs exposed to the risk of injury.

Surgeons from all over the country went to Shanghai, examined the patient, talked with the surgeons concerned and on their return, worked out plans with their colleagues. My hospital in Peking selected a team of surgeons and nurses who would always be available to deal with such cases. We ensured that the necessary instruments and drugs were kept in a state of readiness. We studied the world literature on blood vessel anastomosis and embarked on a series of animal experiments to provide experience in the techniques involved and to answer some unresolved questions. Before long, quite a number of our surgeons could reattach dogs' legs with a fair certainty of success, and we then started experiments on severed rabbits' ears. This was a much more stringent test of surgical technique, for the main blood vessels in a rabbit's ear are considerably finer than a match-stick and the slightest imperfection in technique will result in failure.

We found that we needed finer needles and thread than any then available in China. After explaining our requirements to factories making surgical instruments and synthetic fibres, they produced suitable stainless steel surgical needles and a synthetic fibre of great tensile strength, smooth surface and very small diameter.

In order to increase our accuracy in inserting the stitches, we consulted a technician in an optical equipment factory. He lent us an operating microscope made by a famous German optical firm, but, after using it a few times, we found that although it increased our accuracy, it impeded our movements. The factory technician came to watch us use it and then went back and designed a much superior instrument with a built-in light source and controls that the surgeon could operate with his feet.

Soon we succeeded in reattaching a rabbit's ear.

Not longer after, our first patient arrived. The conditions were not as favourable as they had been with Wang Cung Po for the cut was not clean and there was a good deal of crushing of tissues. But on the other hand, we were fully prepared and had the benefit of Shanghai's experience. The operation went off smoothly and the result was excellent. One reason for our success was that we now knew that in order to avoid swelling of the reattached limb, it was necessary to join up more veins than arteries because, since blood flows through arteries much faster than through veins, if only the same number of veins and arteries are joined up, there is bound to be an accumulation of blood in the part.

We made a colour movie of the operation and, during a visit home in 1965, I showed it to surgical audiences in Britain and elsewhere. A few months after I had shown it in Greece, I had a letter from a Greek surgeon telling me that it had helped him to reattach a youth's arm.

Soon both the medical profession and the general public realized the new possibilities which had opened up, and patients were being flown into the large cities from remote areas. We also started receiving requests for surgeons to assist local doctors in dealing with these cases and we always responded positively.

When patients started coming from far and wide, it became apparent that the time factor was very important. The longer the interval between injury and operation, the smaller the chance of success. Experimental work in the USA had led to the conclusion that an interval of six hours was the maximum and that beyond this, not only was failure inevitable, but operation could be dangerous to life.

Chinese experimenters investigated the effects of refrigeration and found that if the amputated part was kept at a temperature just above freezing point, the permissible interval between amputation and reattachment could be greatly prolonged.

Although not all parts of China have refrigeration apparatus suitable for the transportation of severed limbs, ice-lollies and large thermos bottles are available everywhere and before long patients started arriving with their severed limbs in vacuum bottles surrounded by ice-lollies. Although this is not a very reliable or scientific method, it prolonged the permissible interval considerably. By 1966 a large number of amputated limbs had been successfully reattached and a case was even reported from a remote hospital where the surgeon, lacking suitable needles and suture material, had improvised a surgical needle out of an acupuncture needle and had used human hair in place of silk or nylon thread.

Since then still more experience has been gained and it is no exaggeration to say that such operations are no longer out of the ordinary.

Fingers too

Accidental limb amputations are not very common but finger amputations are. In a busy accident centre such as the one in which I worked in Birmingham, finger amputations are seen every day.

It is therefore not surprising that, following on the successful reattachment of whole limbs, Chinese workers should start to request that their severed fingers be reattached. And it is even less surprising that Chinese surgeons, imbued as they are with a desire to serve the labouring people, should do their best to succeed.

In some respects it is more difficult and in other respects easier to reattach a severed finger than to reattach an entire limb. It is more difficult because the blood vessels are finer, more difficult to handle, more liable to become blocked by blood clot and more liable to go into spasm.

120

It is easier because the soft tissues in a finger are less complicated and less likely to become infected. There are no muscles in a finger and only three tendons as compared with twenty tendons above the wrist. The nerves in a finger are responsible only for sensation, not for movement, and they recover more quickly and more completely than nerves elsewhere.

Surgeons in the Sixth Municipal Hospital in Shanghai failed twenty times before, on 8 January 1966, they had their first success in reattaching a severed finger. Each time they analysed the cause of failure. They tried various devices for joining the blood vessels but eventually they decided that the use of ordinary interrupted sutures inserted with great care and gentleness, was the simplest and best method. They practised unceasingly. During actual operations they used no special aids but the assistant would check up with a magnifying glass and if one stitch was the slightest bit inaccurate, it was removed and replaced. Meticulous post-operative care was of key importance.

To snatch victory from defeat, a surgeon must be prepared to re-operate without delay whenever failure threatens, and to learn to distinguish between the various causes of failure. Some cases were re-operated on three or four times with a total operating time of as much as twenty-four hours before the digit could be pronounced out of danger.

A successful first operation to reattach all four fingers and the thumb took seventeen hours and, on an average, one amputated finger takes four hours.

In the year following their first success, surgeons at the Shanghai Sixth Municipal Hospital saved twenty-four completely and twelve incompletely amputated fingers. I have personally seen many of them and found that the reattached fingers have good sensibility and are used in both skilled and heavy manual work.

Spare-part surgery

Up to the present, this work has been concerned with reattaching the patients' own severed extremities, and though there are still a number of technical problems, these can be solved within a relatively short time.

In the future, another and more exciting prospect will open up. When the immunological problems associated with homografting, that is, with the transfer of living tissue from one individual to another, have been solved, the possibility will arise of changing new limbs for old. Then a new era, the era of spare-part surgery will dawn.

Chinese scientists working in this field may not yet be in sight of victory but I am confident that the factors which have enabled them to climb one peak of science after another, will help them climb this one too. When that happens we shall all be the richer for it.

The common factor

I have described three of a number of fields in which Chinese medical scientists have reached or surpassed the most advanced work done elsewhere.

I think there is a common factor and that is that they closely reflect and are determined by the political system and the political thinking in China. I know that in the West it is customary to draw a sharp distinction between politics and science, and even to deny that there is any intrinsic connection between them, but in China they are manifestly and consciously linked together with politics in the leading position. Here I do not use the word 'politics' in its narrow 'party political' sense but in its wider sense which includes all those factors determining the direction of development of a society.

What is the basis for saying that these three successes reflected and were determined by the political system and current political thinking?

Firstly, all three relied on the conscious use of Marxism-Leninism, the thought of Mao Tse-tung, for the solution of key problems. Marxism-Leninism is, of course, no magic formula which computer-fashion automatically gives the answers to questions. Rather it guides us to the key questions, and by so doing, can decide the difference between success and failure.

Secondly, all three endeavours were characterized by collective, as opposed to competitive work. Within the collective there was no jostling for fame or rewards. Information and experience were disseminated to all who needed them.

Thirdly, the medical workers, the masses of the people and the authorities concerned, encouraged and supported each other. This is particularly obvious in the treatment of burns. China is a poor country, but when I showed the case records of a severe burn treated in my hospital in Peking to a leading British burn expert, he said no other country in the world could afford to devote so many human and material resources to save an ordinary worker.

China can do so because the Party and Government represent the interests of the working people, the source of all wealth, and professional workers have the over-riding duty of serving them. Thus expense, in the narrow pecuniary sense of the word, ceases to be relevant.

Fourthly, and most important of all, the moral qualities which are explicit in the teaching of Mao Tse-tung and which more and more are becoming an integral part of the Chinese people, played a decisive role in ensuring victory. These qualities are exemplified by the tenacity which enables a surgeon to operate for seventeen hours on end and then, the following day, to re-open blood vessels one millimetre in diameter in order to remove blood clot; by the courage that drives a group of twenty-five year old scientists, lacking everything except audacity and confidence, to storm one of the sacred citadels of science; by the sense of whole-hearted service that impels teams of doctors and nurses to sacrifice their leisure, contact with their families, even fresh air and sunshine for weeks at a stretch in order to bring a desperately ill burnt patient back from the brink of the grave.

These are some of the political factors which are inseparable from the successes I have described.

It would be wrong not to make it clear that at every stage and in every way, these political factors of a socialist nature have been opposed by political and ideological factors working in the opposite direction, that there has been a struggle between two lines, a struggle which has been coming to a climax during the Cultural Revolution.

Just as the spokesmen of the conservative and reactionary forces poured cold water on the young scientists who were trying to synthesize insulin, so during the battle for the life of Chiu Tsai Kang, they said that we were trying the impossible, wasting the resources of the state, chasing after the spectacular, etc., etc. When doctors were assembled for consultations, they opposed it saying that we should follow Chairman Mao's policy of self-reliance. But when self-reliant, remote hospitals succeeded in reattaching severed limbs, this was derided as parochialism. This subterfuge of quoting the words of Chairman Mao to oppose the essence of his teaching has become well recognized during the Cultural Revolution and has been dubbed 'waving the Red Flag to oppose the Red Flag'.

China's anti-socialists have consistently used every method to discredit the General Line, the Great Leap and the People's Communes and to bring them to a halt. In the medical field they urged the abandonment of what they called over-ambitious schemes; urged reliance only on experts; advocated the divorce of politics from medicine; urged that material incentives should replace the spirit of service and patriotism; urged that Chinese scientists should be subservient to Western science and opposed the new orientation of medical services towards the countryside.

In short, they opposed all that was new and distinctively socialist and urged a return to old outlooks and old methods which are being discarded by the Chinese people. There were times when the issue seemed to lie in the balance but victory in the Cultural Revolution has ensured that the socialist line of Chairman Mao will win out.

12

Health and the peasants

To understand the present, it is necessary to view it against the past.

China has always been a predominantly agricultural country with four fifths of her people living in the countryside and yet it is no exaggeration to say that before Liberation most of China's peasants had virtually no access to modern medicine and very scant access to traditional medicine. Modern type doctors congregated in the towns, where there was money to be made. Traditional doctors, widely regarded as the highest authorities in all matters pertaining to science and art, were closely linked with the landlords and officials. Many of them lived in the county towns, and their scarcity value in the villages enabled them to charge fees which were beyond the reach of the mass of poor peasants. Their herbal remedies were often very expensive, for it was held to be self-evident that cheap medicines were ineffective in comparison with dear ones.

Some traditional doctors were prepared to visit villagers in their homes without payment, but others demanded a fee and suitable transportation, which, in the area I am familiar with, involved a retinue of guards with either a comfortably saddled mule or donkey, or a sedan chair and bearers. Traditions had to be observed. Custom demanded that a visiting doctor must be wined and dined with an unspecified but clearly understood degree of luxury before seeing the patient. If he had travelled far or if the weather was bad, he had a right to expect hospitality in accordance with his station for as long as he desired. All this was only possible for the landlord class, and ordinary peasants could only call a doctor through the good offices of the landlord. If a peasant reinforced his supplications with adequate material inducements, his landlord might consent to call a doctor, ostensibly to see a member of his own household, but actually to see the peasant. Here too, there were binding unwritten conventions. Things had to be so arranged that it would appear that only because the doctor had an observant eye had he noticed the plight of the patient hovering in the background, and only because he had a compassionate heart, had he consented to treat him. The landlord host, basking in the reflected glory of the doctor, despite a display of custom-decreed protests, would munificently pay his fee. The reckoning came later and might plunge the peasant into debt for many years to come.

In view of these crippling financial and social burdens, it is not surprising that although many traditional doctors developed great skill in diagnosis and treatment and although some unreservedly placed their skill at the service of the people, the peasants looked elsewhere for relief from their suffering.

In many villages, a peasant with a flair for acupuncture or manipulation would gradually acquire a reputation and would be called in to treat the sick. Often he would train his son, who, in turn, would extend his skill by learning to recognize and infuse wild medicinal herbs. Although these village 'doctors' were illiterate and were despised by the professional traditional doctors and although the medicine they practised was crude and rudimentary, they did a certain amount of good and created the social climate for the subsequent training of true peasant doctors.

Superstitious practices were widespread. Witch-doctors, usually unkempt semi-demented women with an awe-inspiring appearance, attributed illness to ghosts, devils and evil spirits which they tried either to exorcize or placate. Placation involved sacrifices of chickens or other luxuries which the poverty-stricken people couldn't afford, while the evil spirits could only be exorcized by incantations and weird antics, which, if they did not frighten the spirits, certainly frightened the patient and the spell-bound onlookers.

Many harmful superstitions were associated with childbirth. In some areas women had to give birth unaided in a shed or outhouse; in others, mother and child were kept in a darkened room for several weeks after delivery; elsewhere, the baby could not be dressed for the first month of life, and after that could only be wrapped in old rags. Ignorant gamps often attended at childbirth, and their practice of biting through the umbilical cord and applying cow-dung to the stump caused many babies to die of tetanus, a disease which, because of its commonness and time of onset, came to be known as 'nine-day illness'.

Poverty and ignorance were reflected in a complete lack of sanitation as a result of which fly and water-borne diseases such as typhoid, cholera, dysentery, took a heavy toll. Worm infestation was practically universal, for untreated human and animal manure was the main and essential soil fertilizer. The people lived on the fringe of starvation and this so lowered their resistance to disease that epidemics carried off thousands every year. The average life expectancy in China in 1935 was stated to be about twenty-eight years. Reliable health statistics for pre-Liberation China are hard to come by but conservative estimates put the crude death rate in times of peace at between thirty and forty per thousand and the infantile mortality rate at between 160 and 170 per thousand live births. The plight of the women and children was bad beyond description. The men had to have what grain there was, to give them strength to work in the fields. The women, especially those who stayed at home to look after the children, ate only thin gruel, grass and leaves. They were so ill-nourished that by the time they reached middle age, they were toothless and decrepit. Many adolescent girls, lacking calcium and vitamin D, developed softening and narrowing of the pelvic bones, so that normal childbirth became either impossible or so dangerous that six to eight per cent of all deaths among women were due to childbirth. Babies were breast-fed for three or four years, for no other food was available. This threw a heavy strain on the mothers, and also resulted in child malnutrition and such vitamin deficiency diseases as rickets and scurvy. There were no preventive inoculations against infectious diseases, and from time to time epidemics of smallpox, diphtheria, whooping cough and meningitis swept through the countryside with devastating results. Lice and poverty went hand in hand, and with them louse-borne diseases such as typhus fever. Military occupation and the licentiousness of the landlords and local gentry spread venereal diseases among the people and no treatment was available. The prevalence of tuberculosis can be gauged from the fact that in 1946 sixty per cent of all applicants for student visas for study abroad were found to be suffering from this disease.

First steps

Such was the public health situation in the rural areas which the People's Government inherited in 1949. It is against this background that subsequent developments have to be seen. I have not exaggerated the enormity of the medical tasks confronting the new regime and its corps of medical workers, but by omission have understated them.

Writing in 1948, Dr Winfield, an American who had spent thirteen years in China, wrote: 'Many of her most common causes of illness and disease are rooted in the very structure of her overcrowded peasant society.'

Since Liberation, the population has increased considerably but the health situation has been transformed, showing that 'over-crowding' was not an important factor.

One of the first steps taken after Liberation was to unite the available medical workers. At this time, the number of modern doctors was certainly much less than one per 100,000 of population, nearly all of them in a few big cities, whereas there were several hundred thousand traditional doctors who enjoyed the confidence of the people. Accordingly, in August 1950, the first National Health Conference was convened and Mao Tse-tung issued a call for unity between traditional and modern doctors.

Whatever they lacked in modern scientific knowledge, there was no doubt that traditional doctors, properly organized, could make a valuable contribution to the protection of the health of the people. It would have been the height of folly and irresponsibility to discard this force before there was something better to replace it. Moreover, as already described, subsequent developments have proved that the modern has a lot to learn from the old and that a combination of the two can open up paths impossible for either alone.

Within two years of Liberation, Chinese volunteers were helping the Koreans to repel US aggression and it became necessary to mobilize the people to protect their health from the dangers arising from the use of germ warfare in Korea. A patriotic health campaign was promoted in response to this need. Tens of millions of people of all ages, guided by sanitary workers who supplied the know-how and the necessary materials, waged a war of extermination against the 'four-pests'—flies, rats, bedbugs and mosquitoes.

The unprecedented success of this campaign has been acknowledged by many Western observers. In many parts of the country, flies were virtually eliminated; an astounding feat in the fly-ridden Orient and one which could only be accomplished by an unusually united and responsive population.

However, the control of flies and other insects requires a long-term, not a temporary campaign, and therefore, after the Korean conflict, the Patriotic Health Campaign remained a permanent part of the Chinese people's war against disease. In the villages it is now closely integrated with the hygiene and sanitary work of the mobile medical teams.

For many years after Liberation, the main effort in developing health services was concentrated in the towns. There were many reasons for this, some of which were valid, while others, during the great scrutiny of the Cultural Revolution, are being re-examined and sharply criticized.

It was urgently necessary to train more doctors, and this necessitated the building of new medical schools and teaching hospitals in the cities. More than fifteen times as many modern doctors graduated between 1949 and 1964 than in the preceding twenty years. In 1963, 25,000 doctors graduated and I believe that China is now turning out more medical workers than any other country in the world. The curriculum for traditional doctors is being standardized and schools of traditional medicine have been established. Medical research has made great progress, and some first class laboratories have been built, equipped and staffed.

At the same time, the rapid development of industry and the corresponding growth in the urban population made it essential to provide medical services for industrial workers and their families. By 1964, the number of urban hospital beds had increased tenfold.

All this explained, or was alleged to explain, the concentration of available medical resources in the towns rather than in the country.

The emphasis changes

The setting up of rural People's Communes throughout the countryside in 1958 radically changed the situation. For the first time in China's history, large-scale collectivization created the political, social and economic conditions which could support a rural system of social security and welfare services.

Notwithstanding their lack of experience, slender resources and a dearth of medical personnel, the majority of the People's Communes established medical clinics and took the first hesitant steps along the road of disease prevention in the countryside.

Then came three bad years during which, chiefly because of exceptionally wide-spread drought and floods, poor harvests were reaped throughout the country. The Chinese people tightened their belts. The system of People's Communes was severely tested, and the way in which it succeeded in withstanding a succession of savage blows showed that it was well suited to Chinese conditions. It enabled the enormous strength of the people to be fully utilized in the fight against natural calamities and it enabled a rational system of distribution to be put into operation.

During these three years, people were short of food, but none starved. They were not elegantly clad, but all had clothing to protect them from the wind and cold. When the lean years passed, the whole nation realized the truth of what Chairman Mao had been saying for years—that agriculture was and must be the foundation of the national economy.

Agriculture must have priority! The countryside must come first!

These slogans swept through China and found concrete expression in many ways. Industry was reorientated to supply chiefly the needs of the countryside. Consumer goods were produced primarily with the interests of the peasants in mind. Machinery and labour power were allocated unstintingly for the construction of gigantic systems of water conservancy to meet the challenge of flood and drought. Priority was given to the manufacture of chemical fertilizer and agricultural tools and machinery. Electrification of the countryside proceeded apace. Tens of thousands of young city intellectuals responded to the call to settle down in the countryside to reinforce the People's Communes and introduce modern science.

Early in 1965, in response to repeated directives from Chairman Mao, a new and revolutionary policy of orientating the health service mainly towards the countryside started to be adopted.

Now, during the storm of the Cultural Revolution, when everything is being re-examined, when past mistakes are being rectified and the reasons for them brought to light, it has become clear that the reason why this policy had not been implemented earlier was opposition to it by the anti-socialist sector of the Party and State apparatus headed by the then head of State, Liu Shao-chi.

During the first two years of the Cultural Revolution, in the North-Eastern province of Hailungkiang alone, no fewer than 8,400 medical workers left the towns and settled in the rural areas.

There is no doubt that the present drive to bring modern health services to China's peasant millions, which is daily gaining in momentum, is no temporary expedient but a long-term policy which serves the needs of today and of tomorrow. It brings health policy into line with the overall national policy of righting the historic wrong whereby those who laboured hardest, and especially the peasants who comprise eighty per cent of the population, got least.

It is a radical change which has significance for the poverty-stricken, disease-ridden people of Asia, Africa and Latin America, and indeed for people everywhere. It reverses the world-wide tendency for doctors to gravitate from the poorer parts of the country to the richer, from the country-side to the towns, and from the poorer parts of the towns to the more affluent parts. All this has been happening in my own country too. In 1965 the 98,000 people in the coal-rich Rhondda valley had only thirty-nine general medical practitioners to look after them, nine of them being above sixty-five years and one over ninety years of age. There is a constant flow of doctors and other scientific workers from England to the United States and from India to England, in each case from the poorer to the richer country.

The new health policy in China will have repercussions throughout the world.

13

Facing the countryside

Since China is a vast country which is emerging very rapidly from a state of extreme backwardness, it is inevitable that there should be unevenness in both the speed and direction of progress.

In order to avoid the dangers of misrepresentation and over-simplification, I confine this chapter to my personal experience of the new rural medical services in a county on the northern fringe of Hopei province. This is one of the poorer parts of China where the terrain is mountainous, communications poor and the climate hard. For more than a decade, it was part of the puppet Japanese state of 'Manchukuo' and it still bears scars of colonial oppression and devastation. Certainly there are many parts of China where things are much better, where the climate is kinder, the terrain more hospitable and where the establishment of a rural health service has made greater progress. Equally certainly, there are other areas which have not yet reached this level. While the situation which I shall describe may not represent conditions throughout China, it does not exaggerate but probably understates the advances which have been made since the Chinese Communist Party formulated its health policy of orientation towards the countryside.

The new policy is being put into effect in a number of different ways, the most important of which is the sending of mobile medical teams from the towns to the countryside.

Mobile medical teams

In April 1965 my hospital in Peking called for volunteers to organize a medical team to serve a rural area a few hundred miles away in northern Hopei. Within six months it comprised 107 nurses, laboratory workers, administrators and doctors of all specialities and levels of seniority. It is intended that in the near future at least one third of the hospital staff shall be working with the mobile team on a rotation basis, and this proportion will increase later. This team serves twelve People's Communes with a total population of about 80,000 persons. It is divided into three medical brigades, each based on a central clinic which serves the surrounding three or four Communes and is responsible for smaller clinics in selected production brigades. Doctors in the small clinics regularly visit every village within a specified area and are available for emergency calls. All the villages are linked by telephone.

The medical brigade centred on the Four Seas clinic, which serves about 15,000 peasants scattered over a large, mountainous areas has a complement of thirty-five, some stationed in the central clinic and the remainder organized into six small groups based in different villages. Most villages can only be reached on foot or by riding donkeys over stony paths.

The members of the small groups in the outlying villages either live together in peasant cottages which also serve as clinics, or they lodge separately with villagers. In either case they usually eat with villagers, paying for meals at a standard rate. When they are travelling round the outlying villages and it is impossible for them to return to base at night, they stay with peasants, sharing the same kang[1] and helping to carry water and collect firewood for the household.

At least once a week, and more often during the busy farming seasons, the medical workers join the peasants in manual labour in the fields.

The usual period of service with the mobile team is one year, all its members are volunteers and a balance is maintained between new graduates and experienced doctors and between the different specialities. Whatever their original speciality, while they are in the countryside, doctors are expected to undertake any kind of medical work. To equip them for their new life and new work, they receive a preparatory course of training before leaving the city.

They get eight days home leave every two months with free transportation and they are paid their normal Peking hospital salaries while in the countryside. Many of them apply to extend their tours of duty but usually this is not possible since their colleagues in Peking are anxious to replace them. Some volunteer to settle down permanently in the countryside; twelve doctors from my hospital have done so since the scheme started eighteen months ago.

In addition to general mobile medical teams, there are also specialized teams according to local needs and resources. In this area, for example, there is a mobile eye, ear, nose, throat and dental team which spends a month in each People's Commune in turn. There is also a birth control team.

SIX TASKS
The mobile medical teams have six tasks:

TASK ONE
The first task is to provide preventive and therapeutic services in the area served and, in accordance with policy, preventive work is given priority. All children are immunized against infectious diseases by a travelling inoculation team which visits the villages whenever primary immunization or 'booster' doses become due. Before Liberation only vaccination against smallpox was available for the rural population and this involved a journey to the county town and the payment of about ten pounds of grain. Now immunization is free and, to express their appreciation and also to encourage the children to regard the doctors as friends rather than enemies, the villagers make the inoculation team's visit a festive occasion, welcome it with drums and cymbals, gaily decorate the cottage where the injections are to be given and congregate to share the fun. If, notwithstanding this psychological preparation, a child objects to the benefits about to be conferred on him, a pock-marked elder is produced for his education and then there is usually no trouble.

Smallpox, typhoid, diphtheria, infantile paralysis and whooping cough have now practically disappeared from this area and recently Chinese medical scientists have developed a method of active immunization against measles which has greatly reduced its incidence and severity. All children receive oral

[1]A kang is a raised platform of brick or baked mud which usually runs the whole length of the room. It is heated by the flue of a stove and serves as a bed.

BCG against tuberculosis and during epidemics, injections are given against encephalitis and infectious meningitis.

Another aspect of preventive work in the countryside is the prevention of water-borne diseases. Drinking water in the villages comes from wells, rivers or springs which can easily be contaminated with disease-producing germs. The first step was to win the active support of the people, for without this nothing could be done. Lectures illustrated by posters and lantern slides were given and a microscope was set up near a contaminated water source so that the peasants could themselves see the germs swimming about in the water. An old Chinese saying holds that one seeing is worth ten thousand hearings. Once they were convinced that they had been swallowing millions of micro-organisms, they co-operated whole-heartedly.

A village near the Four Seas clinic had only one well and outbreaks of intestinal infection there were common. An investigating group from the mobile medical team found that the water was heavily contaminated. The mouth of the well opened at ground level and was surrounded by mud and excreta which was washed into the well whenever it rained. Moreover, as many peasants regretfully affirmed, not a few piglets and chickens had fallen into the well, never to be seen again. The team suggested building a low wall around the mouth of the well, covering it with removable wooden boards and paving the surrounding soil with stone slabs. The peasants agreed and working together with the doctors and nurses, soon had the job done. After this, outbreaks of intestinal infection gradually ceased and a few weeks later the peasants could see that there were no more wriggling germs in the water. Drums and gongs to celebrate victory over the tiny enemy! And the word got around that these young doctors sometimes knew what they were talking about and that it might be worthwhile to listen to their advice.

Nearby Pearl Spring village is so named because of a beneficent spring which supplies it with abundant water even in times of drought or when other villages are ice-bound. It seemed impossible that such crystal clear water could be a source of danger but attacks of diarrhoea and vomiting were common. The cause became clear when mobile team members went to investigate. The spring opened on a hillside a few hundred yards away and to save themselves unnecessary walking, the villagers had led the water down a stone-lined ditch into the village. The trouble was that on this short stretch, children played in the stream, women washed clothes in it and animals drank from it. Inside the village, it flowed into an open pool into which buckets were dipped. Mobile team members calculated that it would cost very little to lead the water through earthenware pipes to a spot where it could fall directly into buckets and when the peasants were convinced that this would be healthier and more convenient, they jointly carried out the necessary work.

Sometimes it is impossible to make water safe at the source and then it must be sterilized after it has been collected. Since this region lacks coal and the accumulation of brush wood is labour consuming, boiling is not practicable and chlorination is often used instead. Water is stored in large earthenware urns and bleaching powder, which is issued free, is added to reach a chlorine concentration of from one per cent to three per cent which sterilizes the water without excessively affecting its taste.

A very important aspect of preventive work concerns the disposal of human and animal excreta. This is not a schistosomiasis area but faeces can spread diseases in three ways. Firstly, by contaminating drinking water it can spread water-borne diseases. Secondly, it can provide a breeding place for flies which carry the germs of dysentery and gastro-enteritis. Thirdly, it can spread hook-worm and round-worm for, if untreated faeces containing worm eggs is used as fertilizer, the crops will be contaminated with eggs which will grow into mature worms after being swallowed. The mobile teams urge the peasants to use leak-proof, covered latrines and they themselves have constructed many prototypes about two feet long, one foot wide and one foot deep, lined with bricks or with stones bound with lime and covered by a wooden board. When the peasants appreciate their advantages, they are widely adopted and in some villages every house now has its own latrine.

When the latrines are emptied the excrement, mixed with animal dung, is treated by a simple process of high-temperature composting. A mixture of equal parts of dung, earth, water and straw is piled into a specially prepared pit in which vertically placed sheaves of maize stalks provide ventilation. Gradually, the temperature of the compost rises high enough to kill harmful worm eggs and make it safe for use as fertilizer. After high temperature composting, the manure becomes lighter in weight and easier to spread while its effectiveness as fertilizer is enhanced.

In the northern mountainous region where I worked, lice elimination is also part of the preventive work carried out by the mobile medical teams, for lice can spread typhus fever. This is one of the activities where the duties of the health workers and of the Patriotic Health Campaign overlap. The mobile team supplies the know-how and the materials while the actual work is carried out by volunteers working under the local committee of the Patriotic Health Campaign. In this region, lice are only a problem in the cold weather when the peasants wear padded clothes and sleep under quilts which are not easily washed. A delousing team equipped with sprayers and a solution lethal to lice, visits every cottage while the peasants are working in the fields and thoroughly sprays the quilts and straw mats covering the kang. The peasants habitually sleep on the heated kang covered by quilts and so the same night the delous-ing team returns and sprays their padded clothing. The procedure is repeated three times at weekly intervals and this greatly reduces the number of lice even if it does not completely eliminate them.

Another example of preventive work is the prevention of goitre, which formerly affected most adults in some villages. The main cause, lack of iodine in the drinking water, has now been remedied by adding an iodine compound to table salt. As a result goitre is now less common and in time it will disappear.

The therapeutic or curative work carried out by the mobile teams takes place at three levels; in the central clinics, in the small village clinics and in the homes of sick villagers.

The Four Seas central clinic, which was completed in May 1966, comprises several single storied brick buildings. It does not yet have electricity or running water but these will soon be laid on. It is linked with the surrounding Com-munes by good roads and receives patients at any time. Very low fees, which can be waived when necessary, are charged and paid into the clinic funds.

Most kinds of blood tests can be carried out and in its first six months, 138 operations including radical excision of tuberculous lesions of the spine, intestinal obstruction, Caesarian section, removal of the gall bladder, hernia and appendicectomy were performed there. A few years before, none of these operations could have been performed in the countryside, the patients would have gone without treatment and many of them would have died.

Although the therapeutic work at the next level, in the small village clinics, is on a modest scale, its value should not be underestimated. These clinics, housed in typical three-room peasant cottages, use one room for clinical examination, one for minor surgery and midwifery, and one as a pharmacy. Patients are seen at any time of the day or night, the staff consisting of three or four doctors and nurses from the mobile medical team and a few traditional doctors. Originally the traditional doctors conducted private practice, directly charging fees for their services. Then they amalgamated to form group practices which were still essentially of a private nature. Next they formed collectives, paid their fees into a common fund and drew fixed salaries. The advent of the mobile team increased the scope of their work but lowered its profitability because the fees charged by the mobile team were much lower than their own. To solve this problem, the mobile team members now also pay their receipts into the common fund of the traditional doctors who, in return, have lowered their charges to the mobile team level. This means, in effect, that a Peking municipal hospital is subsidizing medical services for peasants some hundreds of miles away, for it still pays the salaries of mobile team members. This cannot be a permanent arrangement and the method of remuneration of traditional doctors in the village clinics must undergo further change. One possibility which is being discussed is for the People's Communes to incorporate the village clinics and either pay their medical workers fixed salaries, or enrol them as commune members and allocate them work points in the usual way. The only final solution is a free comprehensive medical service for all, but this is not yet feasible. One of the important lessons of the new health policy is that by relying on the socialist consciousness and enthusiasm of medical workers, and by training local personnel, it is possible in China to improvize a rural health service very cheaply during the course of building up the country. It will not take many years before a comprehensive free health service is available for all.

The third level of therapeutic service is in the villagers' own homes and even in the fields while they are working. This is certainly the most novel and possibly also the most important aspect of therapeutic work in the rural areas. Team members stationed in the cottage clinics are responsible for weekly or twice weekly visits to every village in the neighbourhood. The villagers know the approximate time of the doctor's arrival and with traditional Chinese courtesy wait for him at the entrance to the village. Everybody knows everybody else in these villages and it is not necessary to inquire far to find out who is sick, where he lives and what his symptoms are. As the doctor goes from cottage to cottage he collects an ever-growing retinue of followers and 'advisers', mostly children who give the proceedings a charming atmosphere of informality. The mountain folk are wonderfully generous and warm hearted and though their possessions are meagre they lavish hospitality on their visitors. Many times my pockets have been filled with sunflower seeds and dried dates, delicacies usually reserved for festive occasions. Unlike their brethren in the cities, they never seem to notice that I am a foreigner. On one occasion, after I had sat for some hours chatting on the kang with the village elder, he asked me where I came from since my manner of speech and my appearance seemed somewhat out of the ordinary. Did I come from south China, or was I an overseas Chinese? He was quite amazed when I told him that I was English. 'English!' he said, 'England is a different country! So you're a foreigner! I've never met a foreigner before. They've never been in these parts.'

Thereupon he passed me his pipe and redoubled his efforts to make me eat and drink. When anyone came into the room he would announce proudly 'You'll never guess where this comrade comes from. He's a foreigner—like Bethune.'

This spirit of extreme warm heartedness towards foreigners who support the Chinese revolution is something which I have experienced all over China, and which stands in glaring contrast to allegations of Chinese xenophobia made by ignorant or ill-intentioned persons. The reference to Bethune is one which I often hear and which I find quite embarrassing for Dr Bethune, I should explain, came to China from Canada during the hardest period of the Anti-Japanese war, worked in the front line, eventually sacrificed his life, and for millions of Chinese is the embodiment of proletarian internationalism and of a Communist combination of political, moral and professional qualities.

One might argue that it is not an efficient way of using doctors, when there are so few of them, to let them spend hours tramping from village to village seeing a handful of patients. But that would be a one-sided viewpoint, for it would take no account of the tremendous stimulus to morale which these domiciliary visits give to the peasants who constitute eighty per cent of China's total population. Nor would it allow for the fact that were it otherwise, the doctors could not know how the majority of their fellow countrymen live and work. Nor would it recognize that unless a peasant is really incapacitated, he prefers to put up with aches and pains and go on working rather than take a day off to go and see the doctor. Nor would it take into account the fact that the mobile medical teams are pioneering the rural medical service of the future.

Mobile team members based on the village clinics carry medical boxes with them so that they can dispense medicines on the spot. In the surgical field, at first they performed only minor operations but, with increasing experience, they undertook major emergency operations and later, non-emergency major operations performed in the villagers' own cottages. This saves the peasants much money and trouble and the results have been very good. Although hygienic conditions in the cottages are poor, the post-operative infection rate is certainly no higher and may even be lower than in modern, air-conditioned hospitals. One mobile team of eye surgeons, working in the south of China, performed more than a thousand eye operations without a single case of infection.

134

Elsewhere I describe some operations which have been successfully performed in peasants' cottages in this isolated mountainous region. The examples given could be multiplied many times.

THE SECOND TASK

The second of the six tasks is to train auxiliary medical personnel from among the local people. It is this aspect of their work that I personally consider to hold the key to future advances.

China, like many other countries, needs many more doctors and needs them quickly. China, like *all* other countries, needs doctors who are completely devoted to the welfare of the ordinary people, who understand them, who are not separated from them by barriers of cash or class and who can serve both their immediate and their long-term needs.

I am convinced that after a period of trial and error, the policy of training medical workers from among the local population can meet both of these needs for China.

Since the concept is a new one and is still in an experimental stage, the methods and objectives of training vary greatly from province to province but the objective everywhere is to train one peasant doctor for each production brigade, one volunteer sanitary worker for each production team and enough midwives to ensure that every peasant woman giving birth is helped by a person of some professional competence.

Since there are some seventy thousand People's Communes in China and every Commune is divided into production brigades which are in turn subdivided into production teams, it is clearly intended to train many hundreds of thousands of medical workers.

I shall again write only about my personal experience in one particular area.

Peasant doctors

In the area served by the Four Seas clinic, the training of peasant doctors started in November 1965 after the autumn harvest had been reaped and the grain was safely in the granaries. Each of the thirty-two production brigades in the area held meetings to select candidates for medical training, giving preference to intelligent youths with three years of secondary school education who had shown concern for the collective interests. Only two girls were selected because of a natural reluctance to train people who might leave their villages when they marry. The thirty-two candidates went to Four Seas clinic where they were interviewed by their prospective teachers and they studied there until the following April when they returned to their villages in time for the spring sowing.

Throughout their period of training, emphasis was placed on developing those Communist qualities so stressed by Mao Tse-tung, of selfless service to the people, of limitless responsibility in work and of perseverance in the face of difficulties. The intention was not merely to impart medical knowledge, but to evolve a new kind of socialist-minded rural health worker who would retain the closest links with the peasants and be content to stay permanently in the countryside.

135

For the first two weeks they studied anatomy and physiology, dissected pigs, and attended lectures illustrated by models and lantern slides. After this introductory course they learned the elements of bacteriology and pathology in the mornings and clinical medicine and hygiene in the afternoons. They learnt to identify germs in contaminated water and to recognize the eggs of worm parasites in excreta. They learnt how to make drinking water safe, how to treat night-soil, how to sterilize needles and syringes and how to give injections. They learnt how infectious diseases are spread and how to diagnose them. They accompanied their teacher doctors on their rounds, learnt the use of the stethoscope, how to take a medical history, how to diagnose common diseases and how to detect the signs of serious illness. They examined patients who came to the clinic and discussed their findings with the doctor in charge. They concentrated on a few diseases commonly seen in the neighbourhood, and on the use and dosage of some forty drugs. They memorized fifty acupuncture points and the symptom complexes which they control and they practised the technique of acupuncture. Each student was issued with a well illustrated book specially written for peasant doctors.

They studied hard and enthusiastically. Late at night, they read aloud to each other by the uncertain light of oil lamps, discussing problems and never hesitating to consult their teachers with whom they lived as equals and with whom they shared the day-to-day household chores, in addition to nursing the patients.

As the winter went by and the frozen streams began to thaw, the students gained in confidence and initiative. They took it in turns to be on night duty, welcoming patients who came from afar with a hot drink and a friendly greeting and making a preliminary examination before calling the doctor.

Five months is a very short time in which to learn the rudiments of medicine but these students learnt more in five months than I would have thought possible. They learnt fast because their studies were practical and combined theory with practice, because they were determined to justify the trust put in them by their own folk and because, although young, they were mature working men, disciplined and capable.

While studying, they were credited with the number of work points which they would have earned if they had remained in their villages. Tuition and accommodation were free, they brought grain with them and went home for more when necessary.

In the spring when they returned to their brigades, they were issued with medical boxes, resumed work in the fields, but also looked after the health of their fellow peasants. Their medical work was unpaid but if it resulted in a loss of work points, these were made up. They supplied drugs at cost price, using the money to replenish their stocks and getting more when needed from the brigade cashier.

I spent many hours talking, walking and working with Wang Sheng-li, a twenty-eight year old peasant doctor in training. He is a slightly built, intelligent, earnest young man who models himself on Dr Bethune. He told me that he was determined to master his new profession and to use his skill unstintingly in the service of his fellow peasants. He wore a Red Guard armlet and described how the Cultural Revolution in his village was sweeping

136

away superstition and other obstacles to the advance of socialism, changing bad habits and replacing them by beneficial ones. The old custom of giving mothers nothing to eat but gruel for three months after childbirth had been criticized and now mothers were given eggs, fish and bean-curd. A nearby temple had been stripped of unsuitable paintings and converted into a children's nursery. He was intensely interested in politics, read the news-papers avidly, listened to the radio and was never without his little red book of quotations from the writings of Mao Tse-tung which he cited frequently and aptly.

I joined him and Dr Chen, a consultant physician and one of Wang's teachers from the previous winter, on their weekly round of patients. Young Wang told Dr Chen about his diagnosis and treatment and listened eagerly to his comments. Impressed by the accuracy of Wang's observations, I asked him to tell me about his recent surgical experiences. He thought for a moment and then told me of four surgical emergencies he had dealt with in the last few weeks.

'The first one,' he said, 'was Old Gao, a carpenter over in Ten Family Inn village. His wife telephoned to say that a wooden chest which he had been making had fallen on him a few hours before and that he seemed to be in a bad way. I went over to see him and found him groaning and moaning and rolling all over the kang. I couldn't count his pulse rate since I had gone straight from the fields and didn't have my watch with me but it was certainly faster than mine and I had been hurrying. His belly was as hard as a board. I always have my medical box with me so I got out my blood pressure apparatus and measured his blood pressure. As far as I could make out, the high pressure was only 60 m.m. but I'm not very good at measuring the blood pressure, and I might have been wrong. Then I listened to his belly with my stethoscope. I knew that I should hear some gurgling noises showing that the intestines were working normally but I couldn't hear a thing. That made me think that he must have burst something inside his belly and that the best thing to do was to get him to the Four Seas clinic as quickly as possible. It's not very far and Old Gao's son and myself took turns at carrying him on our backs, but by the time we had gone half way, he was shouting that he couldn't stand the pain so I gave him an injection of pain killer. The pain killer worked well and we got to Four Seas before sunset.'

Dr Chen took up the story. 'We operated on him that night and found that young Wang was quite right. He had torn a hole in his large intestine and there was nearly a pint of blood in the abdomen. It might have been better if Wang had called us out rather than bring Old Gao in because although it's not very far, it's a long way for a sick man and it's rough going. Anyway, he did very well and is back at work now.'

The peasant doctor told me about his next case. 'Strangely enough, my next emergency was from the same village. This time it was Old Liu, the team leader. He's always having attacks of diarrhoea because he was on the Long March[1] and lived on tree bark, grass and soup made of boiled leather and such like for nearly a year and that spoiled his stomach. He looked a bit drawn

[1] The epoch-making 8,000 mile march of the Chinese Red Army from South-East to North-West China in 1934-5.

137

but he was still working, so I gave him some sulpha tablets which usually do the trick. But a few days later he was still running to the latrine five or six times a day and he looked definitely weaker. As it happened the next day was Dr Chen's day to visit Ten Family Inn and Dr Chen gave him some syntomycin tablets and told him to stay on the kang and drink plenty of boiled water with sugar and salt added to it. But he got worse and worse and a couple of days later they telephoned and said that he was vomiting everything and was not very clear in his mind. That really frightened me, for if any person is usually clear in his mind it's Old Liu who has been in the Party since he was a nipper. I more or less ran all the way and found him semi-conscious, his skin all shrivelled and dry and his breath smelling very bad. He'd only passed about a cupful of urine since the previous night and it was deep yellow in colour.

'I 'phoned up Dr Chen and he told me to bring him in to the clinic right away. So we lifted a door off its hinges to serve as a stretcher and two of us prepared to carry him in. We'd learnt from our experience with Old Gao that it's very uncomfortable for a sick man to be carried on the back and Old Liu was really sick.

'Before we set off I thought to myself since he needs fluid and can't drink it, why not give it directly into his vein? I had a bottle of sterile saline with me and I had seen it done several times when I was learning this job in Four Seas. So I fixed him up with an intravenous drip and we let it run in slowly as we carried him to Four Seas. Of course, we needed a third person to hold up the bottle and that made it a bit difficult on the narrow paths, but the drip was still running when we arrived.'

'I really blame myself for not having gone out there,' said Dr Chen. 'He was seriously dehydrated and it's a good thing that young Wang gave him that intravenous drip which contributed to his quick recovery. I had seen him only two days before and I didn't expect him to deteriorate so rapidly.'

The third emergency was a typical case of acute appendicitis in a girl of fifteen.

'The diagnosis was easy this time,' said the peasant doctor. 'She had been perfectly well in the morning, in the afternoon she suddenly had cramp-like pains in the belly, and half an hour later she vomited. This was in my own village and her mother came running out to the field where I was working to fetch me. Her tongue was furred, she had a little fever and when I pressed below and to the right of the navel she winced with pain. I looked up "appendicitis" in my medical book and it fitted perfectly. I 'phoned up the clinic, they sent out a surgical team and by sunset they had removed her appendix. I watched the operation and then the doctors showed me the appendix. It was red and swollen and turning yellow at the tip. When they cut it open it was full of pus. They said it would have burst within a few hours.

'The fourth case is hardly worth talking about,' he said. 'The patient lives very near. We can go and see him if you like.' We walked to a nearby cottage and were greeted by a boy with a recent scar going nearly all round the tip of his nose. 'He was using a sickle for the first time,' young Wang explained, 'and he nearly cut his nose off. It was only joined on by a narrow strip of skin and I didn't know whether it could survive. But he'd have looked very odd without a nose so I decided to give him a chance and sew it back. By good luck it has turned out all right.'

The boy's mother intervened. 'I don't call it good luck,' she said. 'It's skill —that's what it is. He stitched that nose back as though he were doing embroidery. We're proud of our young peasant doctor and grateful to him.'

Young Wang was embarrassed. 'There's no need to be grateful to me,' he muttered. 'I'm grateful to all of you. You've given me a chance to do two jobs instead of one and naturally I want to do them as well as I can.'

I went home with him and was surprised to find that he was married and already had two young children. A picture of Dr Bethune was pinned on the wall and beneath it there was a quotation from Chairman Mao calling upon the Chinese people to learn from Bethune's Communist spirit of proletarian internationalism, his selflessness, his warm-heartedness and his sense of responsibility in his work.

The provisional plan is for peasant doctors to have at least three periods of full-time teaching at yearly intervals. As I write, the land is again in the grip of winter and the thirty-two peasant doctors who started their training last year have reassembled at the Four Seas 'medical school' for their second course of study.

The method of study is different from what it was last year because the teachers now have experience in training peasant doctors and because the requirements of the students are different.

Last year they studied only commonly seen diseases, but this year they systematically study all the diseases of particular organs. For example, last year when learning about lung diseases, they only studied bronchitis, emphysema and asthma while this year they are learning about pneumonia, pleurisy, tuberculosis and lung cancer.

Last year they studied anatomy and physiology as a whole in a short, concentrated, superficial course. This year they are re-studying it in relation to diseases of particular organs. When they study lung diseases, they also revise and deepen their knowledge of the anatomy and physiology of the lungs.

Last year diseases were studied at random; this year they are grouped together according to specialities such as medicine, surgery, gynaecology, ophthalmology.

Last year it was not always possible to find actual patients to illustrate their theoretical studies, but this year their teachers know where to find examples of diseases related to lectures given that day.

This year the practical work is conducted mostly in the students' own villages but the students also visit Peking's teaching hospitals and see advanced medical techniques in use. Although it will be many years before these village doctors have access to the latest medical techniques, it is valuable for them to have some knowledge of the level which one day they must reach and surpass.

I know that some educationalists in the West view this kind of experiment with apprehension and talk of the dangers of 'lowering standards'. They should realize that before Liberation, when the handful of medical students in the Rockefeller-endowed Peking Union Medical College had higher standards and a longer course of study than medical students in England or America, this did not benefit the Chinese peasants, for the overwhelming majority of them enjoyed no medical services of any kind. Chairman Mao quotes an old Chinese saying to the effect that what is needed is not more flowers embroidered on the brocade but fuel in snowy weather.

The training of peasant doctors makes it possible not only to increase rapidly the available medical personnel in China's countryside, but also, in the long term, to produce a better type of doctor than orthodox methods of training can do. It is much more than a temporary expedient. Whatever gaps a peasant doctor may have in his medical knowledge can be made good as he gains experience or by joining refresher courses in city hospitals. His uniquely valuable characteristic is his closeness to his patients. They are his own folk and there is mutual trust and confidence between them. The results of his work are constantly tested in practice in such a way that he can learn immediately both from success and failure. He is both a peasant and a doctor and cannot sink into narrow professionalism or become mentally divorced from the people he serves.

In addition to training peasant doctors, the mobile teams also train sanitary workers and midwives. The former, who receive two weeks' training in basic first-aid and sanitary work, continue to work mainly as peasants but are also available for minor injuries and for ensuring that the water protection and night-soil disposal procedures initiated by the mobile teams are maintained and extended. They are issued with first-aid materials and a few drugs for minor ailments.

The latter are usually village girls in their twenties, although some are older and are themselves mothers. They are given a few weeks' practical and theoretical instruction in the principles of midwifery and accompany the doctors when they conduct ante-natal examinations and deliveries. Their duties are to anticipate difficulties in childbirth by regular ante-natal examinations and to assist women who have previously had normal deliveries. In case of difficulty, they call on the mobile team for help. Although they cannot become expert midwives after a few weeks' training, that can be remedied by further experience and repeated courses. They are undeniably a big improvement on the ignorant, unhygienic gamps whom they replace. I spoke to several mothers who had been delivered by these newly trained midwives and they were well satisfied. One of them said, 'Childbirth used to be a dangerous ordeal but now we approach it with a light heart, knowing that we and our babies will survive.' The population in her village had doubled since Liberation because of the phenomenal reduction in infantile and maternal mortality and the complete disappearance of the tragic necessity, for so long imposed by poverty and hunger, of doing away with baby girls at birth.

THE THIRD TASK

The third task is to make the Party's policy of planned parenthood become a reality in the Chinese countryside.

This is not a nation-wide policy, for some national minority areas such as Tibet, Inner Mongolia and parts of Yunnan are, as a result of centuries of poverty, disease, and oppression, dangerously underpopulated. Here the policy is to improve conditions and gradually to build up the population.

140

To make planned parenthood available to all, it is necessary first to educate the people to understand its advantages and secondly to provide them with the means of achieving it. The mobile teams carry out both these tasks.

I attended an evening lecture on hygiene and birth-control illustrated by an old-style magic lantern using a pressurized paraffin lamp. The village hall was packed and, although children were nominally excluded, they couldn't resist the fascination of the brightly lit coloured lantern slides. At first they peered through the windows and then, as the pressure on window space grew, they infiltrated into the hall until they became a majority of the audience.

After dealing with such mundane subjects as night-soil disposal, fly control and food protection, the speaker, a doctor from the mobile team, described the anatomy and physiology of the male and female organs of reproduction. An animated filmstrip showed the process of penetration of the sperm into the ovum and a gasp of astonishment greeted the spectacle of the fertilized ovum dividing and re-dividing until it looked first like a raspberry and then like a curled-up tadpole.

Then he described various methods of contraception, discussed their advantages and disadvantages and passed round contraceptive appliances for inspection. At this point the children lost interest and filed out, admonished by their parents to go straight home.

He spoke of the advantages of planned parenthood, showing that limitation of families to two or three children was in the interests of the children, of their parents and of the country; that mothers would be better able to look after their children; that schools would be less crowded; that mothers would be able to play a bigger part in producing wealth for the benefit of all; and that mother and child would be healthier and happier.

He urged the women to discuss it among themselves and with their husbands.

When he had finished, the barrage of questions showed that the women were deeply interested in the new possibilities opening up for them.

Subsequently, I asked many village women what they thought of family planning and their answers revealed two conflicting, but perfectly understandable, trends. One was that in the past they had been too poor to raise children, many had died at birth or starved to death and those who survived had gone hungry, naked and unlettered. Now that there was food and schools for all, and life was pleasant and secure, why should they restrict their families? This view was warmly supported by grandparents steeped in the Confucian tradition that many grandchildren brought them honour, prosperity and social security.

The other trend was to welcome the idea of planned parenthood and to appreciate its advantages but sometimes to doubt whether it was possible.

The propagandists first try to win the support of the peasants' own organizations, especially the women's organizations, for once this has been done the idea usually gains acceptance.

The means of contraception are provided free by the State and specialized family planning mobile teams have been organized for propaganda and instruction in the technique of birth-control. Many methods are in use but none are ideal. A large-scale trial of the contraceptive pill is in progress but it is too early to be certain that it is free from risk. The intra-uterine device is fairly satisfactory in towns but in the countryside, among women who do heavy manual labour, it has been found to have disadvantages.

Research work, propaganda and practical work go hand in hand and I am sure that, before long, Chinese women in town and countryside will be able to control the size and spacing of their families according to their wishes.

THE FOURTH TASK

The fourth task is to co-operate with and raise the level of the medical services which existed in the countryside before the mobile teams arrived on the scene.

Developments in the Four Seas Clinic illustrate this. The clinic was established by the county government in 1952 with a staff of one traditional doctor and one pharmacist. Later they were joined by other traditional and middle-grade doctors but they were professionally isolated and their accommodation and equipment were poor. The advent of highly-trained members of the mobile team, and of doctors from Peking who have settled down in the countryside, has made an enormous advance possible. They work together as a team, learning from each other and consulting on difficult problems. The newcomers contribute their knowledge of modern medicine and the original clinic members their knowledge of local conditions and of traditional remedies. The old shacks in which they originally worked have been replaced by a large brick building with accommodation for twenty-five patients, an operating room, an out-patient department, a laboratory where biochemical and blood-tests can be carried out and a library of medical books and journals. It has become, in effect, a small modern rural hospital serving fifteen thousand people.

The same kind of progress, on a more modest scale, can be seen in the little village clinics. The old fee-paying system and the last vestiges of private practice are disappearing. Even tiny clinics like the one in Pearl Spring village have a microscope and apparatus for blood-testing. The original staff there exchange experiences with their colleagues from Peking and refresher courses are arranged for them in leading Peking hospitals.

THE FIFTH TASK

The fifth task is to co-operate with and assist the Patriotic Health Campaign, a mass movement which originally concentrated on eliminating flies, bedbugs, rats and mosquitoes. Under the stimulus of the mobile medical teams, its work now includes lice elimination, water control, food protection and the safe disposal of night-soil. In several villages, Patriotic Health Campaign activists, working in co-operation with mobile medical team members, have used simple, indigenous methods to install running water systems and bath houses. Through the Patriotic Health Campaign, the mobile teams are linked directly with the villagers.

THE SIXTH TASK

The sixth task is for members of the mobile medical teams to utilize the opportunity of a year in the countryside, in close contact with the peasants, to deepen their understanding of the labouring people, and to change their thinking in such a way that they fit better into the new society and become more effective in building socialism.

Though this task is less concrete than the other five, an understanding of it is one of the keys to understanding New China.

A basic tenet of Marxism is that the thinking of people and their moral values are determined by the kind of society in which they live and by their status in that society.

It is sometimes assumed that the moral values of one's own day and age have, with slight modifications, always existed; that they are inborn, part of 'human nature', fixed and unchangeable. However, a backward glance shows that this is not so.

In ancient Greece, many slave owners doubtless considered themselves to be enlightened and humane men. They may well have been so according to the standards of their time, but time moved on, society changed and with it men's thinking, so that today slavery is viewed with abhorrence.

In European feudal society, the ruling class considered it right and proper not only that peasants should till their fields, but that they should be serfs tied to their lord's land and, in many places, that the lord should have the right of the first night. Few would defend these rights today.

The capitalist society, in which I was born and bred, fosters the conviction that it is a law of nature that some should live off the labour of others, that some should be rich and some poor, that some should own factories and hire others to work in them, that black people should toil to keep white people in luxury, that the driving force in society should be self-interest.

What slave society, feudal society and capitalist society have in common is that the dominant world outlook in each of them is selfishness.

When the revolution triumphed in 1949 and China started to build socialism, it was relatively easy to change the economic structure of society. But the cataclysmic upheaval by which one class overthrew another was merely the first step on the long road to the society of the future. There remained the much more difficult and protracted task of changing the standpoint, thinking, morals and habits of millions of people so that much of what had seemed 'natural' in the old society would seem unnatural and hateful in the new, and what had seemed impossible in the old society would become desirable and entirely possible in the new.

This process of change, known in China as ideological remoulding, is difficult for everyone but especially so for those who in the old society were accustomed to leading a soft life and enjoying special privileges.

Two thousand years of feudalism in China implanted a deep-rooted contempt for the unlettered peasants in the minds of the intellectuals.

Mao Tse-tung, recalling his own student days, wrote: 'I began life as a student and at school acquired the ways of a student. . . . At that time I felt that intellectuals were the only clean people in the world, while in comparison workers and peasants were dirty. I did not mind wearing the clothes of other intellectuals, believing them clean, but I would not put on clothes belonging to a worker or peasant, believing them dirty. But after I became a revolutionary and lived with workers and peasants . . . I came to know them well . . .

I came to feel that . . . in the last analysis the workers and peasants were the cleanest people, even though their hands were soiled and their feet smeared with cow-dung. . . .'[1]

The sixth task given to the mobile medical teams is, by mixing closely with the labouring people and sharing in their struggles for a better life, to initiate a similar change in their own thinking, so that they can take the first step towards ideological remoulding.

Most of China's doctors and nurses have had little or no contact with peasants. When I joined a mobile team myself, I expected that the process of adjustment from the soft city life to the hard life of the villages would be difficult for them. But I was often surprised to see how quickly my colleagues settled down. Within a few short weeks most of them were enjoying enormous meals of coarse grain which they would never have looked at in Peking, participating enthusiastically in heavy manual labour and feeling thoroughly at home with the peasants. I expressed my surprise to a rather pampered young woman doctor whose airs and graces had earned her the doubtful title of 'Shanghai miss'. She said, 'Yes—I'm surprised too. Before I came down here I thought I'd never be able to live on millet. It's so hard and my stomach has always been delicate. But funnily enough it seems to agree with me. For the first few weeks, life here was really very difficult. The brick kangs were terribly hard to sleep on, I had a horror of lice, the latrines disgusted me and I hated the idea of eating from the same bowl as the peasants. Now I have got used to all these things. I sleep much more soundly than in Peking, lice are nothing to be afraid of and the peasants are so kind and generous that I feel ashamed of my squeamishness. After all, why should I be so choosy? These peasants work from dawn to dusk almost every day of the year producing food for all of us. They don't make a song and dance about it. They are unselfish and are happy to be making their contribution to our country. Now that I have got used to living in the countryside, my heart seems to be warmer, the paths seem broader and the meals more appetizing than any I have eaten before.'

A pretty young nurse with a fringe brushing her eyebrows asked me in a confidential tone if I would help her out of a minor difficulty. 'You see,' she said, 'when I came down here, I brought some slabs of chocolate with me in case I just couldn't eat this peasant food and starved. Now I don't know what to do with it. I'd be ashamed to eat it myself, the children here won't accept it, I can't bring myself to offer it to the peasants, I won't waste it by throwing it away and if I just keep it in my suitcase, it will melt and spoil my clothes. Will you please take it back to Peking with you when you go?'

In one tiny village which I visited, the mobile team members wanted to give me a good fish supper, so they spent hours fishing in a mountain stream but without success. As dusk was falling, they disconsolately prepared to leave, expecting that we would have to eat the usual millet and pickles. A peasant, who had been watching, asked them why they were so anxious to catch fish since, after all, it wasn't a holiday. They explained that a foreign guest had come and they didn't like to offer him plain fare. 'I'll catch some fish for you,'

[1] Yenan Forum on Art and Literature. Mao Tse-tung. *Selected Works. Vol. III. p.* 73.

said the peasant and soon he had landed three little fish and a river turtle weighing nearly two pounds. They were delighted and urged the peasant to accept some money for the turtle, which is an expensive delicacy. He was deeply offended at the suggestion. 'Please don't talk such nonsense,' he said. 'It sounds too much like the old days when money meant everything. But since you probably don't know how to cook turtle, if you like I'll come and cook it for you.'

He did so and we enjoyed a good meal and spent a pleasant evening together.

Nurse Liu, who had been in charge of a ward in Peking before taking a special course of study to equip her for medical work in the countryside, told me of an incident. 'In Peking,' she said, 'I was called Nurse Liu but here the peasants call me Doctor Liu and the first time I heard it I felt very pleased and swelled with pride. Without noticing it, I gradually assumed the airs which I thought were appropriate for a doctor. One day a peasant with an infected foot came to see me. I told him to rest in bed and gave him an injection of penicillin and a lotion to paint on the foot. Next time I saw him, the foot was much worse. I asked him if he had been resting but he replied that he didn't think I understood his case and he had applied soya sauce to his foot. I felt very resentful, told him he could do what he liked and went off in a huff. However, I had a nagging feeling that perhaps I wasn't doing the right thing and after some days I went back to see him again. There was now a large ulcer on the foot and I learned that he had used a corrosive antiseptic. When I told him he must rest and have injections, he asked me whether I thought a dressing of mashed wild apricots would do the trick. I slammed the door in a fury and walked out. Outside, I met the brigade leader who told me that the reason why the patient had no confidence in me was that, at the height of the busy season, I had airily told him to rest without finding out whether it would be reasonable for him to do so, and, moreover, I had given him an injection of penicillin without a word of explanation just as though he had been a dumb animal.

'I felt rather ashamed and after that I visited him every day until the foot was better. When I thought about it later, I realized how high and mighty I had been with him. When his foot got worse, I had wanted him to beg for forgiveness so that I could be charitable and big-hearted. Actually it was he who was big-hearted for he insisted on working, not for his own sake but for the good of the collective.'

Dr Wang, an overseas Chinese from Indonesia, told me about an outbreak of impetigo of the scalp among children in the village where he was stationed. 'Quite a number of children were affected,' he said, 'so I issued penicillin ointment to the mothers and told them to apply it three times a day. However, the disease continued to spread and I discovered that most of the mothers were out working in the fields and that they were not applying the ointment regularly. They had told the children to rub it in but the youngsters couldn't do it thoroughly. So I applied it myself and they soon got better. Before I came to the countryside, I would have considered it beneath my dignity to spend my time rubbing ointment into children's heads. But here it's just a division of labour. The mothers work in the fields to produce food for us all

145

and I, if I am to be fully responsible, as Dr Bethune was, should personally make sure that their children are properly treated.'

Another doctor told me of a bitter lesson he had learned when he had treated a little boy suffering from meningitis. 'When I arrived at the cottage, the parents were overjoyed,' he said. 'They looked on me as a saviour and I felt like one. I assured them that I would soon have their son out of danger but, in spite of working all night, he died very early the next morning. I didn't know what to say to the parents. On the one hand I wanted to console them, but on the other hand I wanted to shield myself. After a mental struggle I decided to tell them that they had called me too late. Just then they came into the room and saw that their child was dead. They were terribly distressed but without hesitation they took me by the arm and started consoling me, telling me that I had worked very hard and had done my best and that I shouldn't take it too hard. I felt so ashamed that tears ran down my cheeks. You see, we doctors are always concerned about our reputations and, although we do the best we can for our patients, we don't really feel that we are from the same family. But these peasants regard us in the same way as they do their own family. They consoled me when their own child died but I was prepared to tell them that they had called me too late. Here in the countryside we treat their physical ailments and they, without knowing it, treat our ideological ailments.'

I would not like to give the impression that ideological remoulding, in the sense in which the Chinese use the word, is an easy process which can be accomplished by reading books, by solitary introspection, by generating a surfeit of good intentions or by roughing it in the countryside for a year or two.

On the contrary, it is a life-long process which, above all, necessitates identification with the struggles of the labouring people to transform the world.

Some mobile team members who seem to make progress while they are in the countryside relapse when they return to the towns. Others never really succeed in learning to 'talk the same language and breathe the same air' as the peasants; they regard their sojourn in the villages as a penance to be endured in the interests of their future.

But, taken by and large, the great majority benefit considerably. They get to know and to like the peasants; become more desirous of serving them wholeheartedly and better able to do so; they start to get rid of their selfishness, their competitiveness and their feelings of superiority.

They start to become the kind of socialist-minded, versatile, resourceful medical worker which China needs in hundreds of thousands.

The sixth task of the mobile medical team is, therefore, the key to the accomplishment of the other five.

14

The soldier's wife

She arrived at the clinic about half an hour before me, having come from across the new concrete bridge, from the range of hills which stretch as far south as the Great Wall. She had come by horse-drawn cart, lying on the floor on a bale of straw, covered by a cotton quilt, her head cradled in her husband's lap. Involuntarily, despite her iron will, she had groaned with pain whenever the cart jolted over a boulder or slithered into a ditch.

I had walked in from the north, tired and dusty after tramping for nearly a week from village to tiny village, hidden in valleys between jagged hills. I was glad to be back and luxuriated at the prospect of eating hot tasty food and lying on a straw mattress.

While I was washing my feet, the young clinic doctor, whom I had helped to train ever since he had graduated six or seven years before, came in.

'I know you are tired, but I'd like you to see a patient who was brought in half an hour ago.'

She lay on a trestle bed, her skin pale beneath the sunburn and of a curiously fine texture, uncommon among the mountain folk. Her cheekbones were prominent. Her breathing was rapid and shallow and her nostrils dilated slightly every time she breathed in.

The young doctor told me the medical history. She had been riding a donkey, sitting sideways on its buttocks, her hands in her sleeves for warmth, when it stumbled and she had fallen hitting her neck against a stone. She had not lost consciousness but had felt a sudden pain in the neck and all four limbs had become paralyzed and numb.

She was thirty-eight years old. Her husband, a tall, gaunt peasant in a padded jacket, hovered in the background, his eyes eloquent with anxiety, as I examined her. The neck muscles stood out indicating that they were guarding a deep injury. There was a slight swelling in the neck and, as she breathed, I could hear a whistling noise. Her arms and legs were paralyzed and none of the normal reflexes were present. The muscles between the ribs were also paralyzed and she relied entirely on her diaphragm to pump air in and out of the lungs. When she coughed the abdomen became more prominent instead of being drawn in to help in the sudden expulsion of air, and this showed that the abdominal muscles too were paralyzed. I tested the sensibility of her skin and found that she had no feeling in the arms and legs or on the trunk below the level of the second rib.

Without disturbing her head, I slipped my hand behind her neck and pressed gently with my fingertips. At the level of the fourth vertebra she winced with pain. She had broken her neck.

The young doctor and I discussed the case. It was obvious that she had injured the spinal cord at the level of the fourth vertebra in the neck, but many other aspects were not yet clear. Had the spinal cord been completely severed or only bruised? If the former, then the outlook was very bad for the paralysis would never recover. If the latter, then with correct treatment she had a chance of recovery. Only time in combination with proper treatment would tell. What was the nature of the bone injury? Was it a fracture of the spine, or a dislocation, or a combination of both? An X-ray would answer that question—if we had an X-ray machine and electricity to operate it. We had neither. Was there pressure on the spinal cord in the neck? If so, we would have to operate, and operate quickly, in order to relieve it and give the delicate spinal cord a chance to recover.

We could find out whether there was pressure by inserting a hollow needle into the fluid surrounding the lower part of the spinal cord and then gently squeezing the neck. In a normal person this causes the brain to swell and, as a result, the pressure of the fluid surrounding the brain and spinal cord rises, but if there were an obstruction in the neck, the pressure wave would be unable to get past it and so there would be no increase in pressure around the lower part of the spinal cord.

My colleague inserted the needle, attached a glass manometer to it and watched the fluid rise until it became stationary at a pressure of 90 m.m. Then I squeezed her neck. Immediately the fluid level in the manometer started to rise again and within ten seconds it had risen by 60 m.m. The test was negative; there was no pressure on the spinal cord and no need to perform emergency surgery.

'I'm glad we need not operate,' said my colleague, 'spinal cord operations are difficult and dangerous, even in well-equipped operating rooms and no one could say that we are well equipped here. How shall we treat her?'

'You know as well as I do,' I said. 'We've seen many such cases together. First she needs an X-ray to tell us precisely what is wrong with the bone structure of the neck and then she needs traction applied directly to the skull to pull the neck into proper alignment, protect the spinal cord from further injury and give the injured tissues a chance to heal. The traction should be continued for about four weeks and then the head and neck should be immobilized in a plaster jacket for about three months. By that time, it will be safe to allow her to move her neck and we shall know how much recovery to expect in the spinal cord.'

'Yes,' he said. 'In Peking you often told us about the treatment of spinal injuries. The trouble is that we are not in Peking. We cannot X-ray her here and we cannot apply skull traction since we haven't got the apparatus. What shall we do?'

More or less automatically I replied that in that case we would have to telephone for an ambulance and send her to the hospital in the county town.

The apparatus for applying continuous traction to the skull is a rather complex and specialized piece of equipment which is hardly possible to improvise. It is like a miniature ice-tongs, the spikes of which fit into holes drilled in the skull bones and the distance between the spikes is controlled by a screw. Traction is applied directly to the skull by attaching a cord to the tongs, passing it over a pulley and suspending a weight from it. With this apparatus it is possible to apply a strong, continuous, painless pull for several weeks which corrects displacement and ensures healing in good position.

The young doctor went to telephone but came back dejected. 'They haven't any skull traction apparatus. They say we should send her to Peking.

I'm afraid the ambulance journey will be very expensive, maybe more than they can afford to pay.'

We broke the news to her husband and he gulped miserably. 'Send her all the way to Peking!' he said, aghast. 'That would throw a tremendous strain on our brigade. We're only a small brigade. Our land is mountainous and arid. For three years running the spring rains were late and we reaped poor crops. Our funds fell very low and we're only just starting to recover. This year we planned to install two electric pumps and buy a husking machine.

'I know they'll raise the money if it's necessary, for they love my wife. They'd all gladly empty their pockets for her. I would do anything in the world for her. But an ambulance to Peking! That would set our brigade back a full year!'

His mate grasped his arm. 'Don't worry about that now. The important thing is to get your wife well again. Do whatever the doctors suggest. I'm sure they understand the position, and won't send her to Peking unless it's really essential. In the meantime, I'll go back to the brigade and tell them about it.' They silently shook hands and he was off.

We walked over to the kitchen to get our evening meal and I asked him whether his wife was a local woman, for she looked different and spoke differently from the local people. He hesitated, seemingly unwilling to reply. Then he told me that she came from Hunan province in south China, that she was the only 'foreigner' in these parts.

We ate in silence and then he suddenly turned to me, gripped my arm fiercely and told me about his wife. 'I married her in Hunan. I was born a few miles from here in the village where we live now, but she was born far away in the soft, warm South. I joined the Eighth Route Army as a lad, ran past the Japanese sentries and up into the hills to find the Red Army. The Army became my father and mother. I grew to be a man in the Army. I fought through the length and breadth of China and when the mainland was liberated I was demobilized. At that time I was in Hunan and I was in no hurry to come back to these parts. Hunan was fine—they call it a land of rice and fish. I farmed the land and rested after the hard years of fighting. I met a beautiful girl, full of youth and energy and optimism. We married and she smoothed away the creases of my suffering and gave me back my youth.

'Life was good in Hunan. Then I started getting letters from my home village asking me when I was coming home. There was so much to be done and so few to do it. The Japanese had burnt everything and then, just when they were rebuilding, the Kuomintang and the war lords came back and burnt it all again. Now there were houses to be built, land to be opened up, wells to be sunk, trees to be planted, countless jobs to be done. Now that the land at last belonged to the people, the people had to heal the scars of war. They said that since I had been in the Liberation Army I must be a skilled man and they needed me. When was I coming home?

'Their letters started a gnawing pain in my heart. Of course they were right! My father had died defending our poor village. Countless fine comrades had died, driving out the invaders and regaining the land for the people! What right had I to spend my days down there in gentle Hunan, eating fine rice and laughing with my wife while my kinsfolk were rebuilding on the ashes of the past? Wasn't it like running away, like deserting in the face of difficulties?

149

'I made up my mind to go back. But my wife had never felt the northern winds, had never eaten the coarse grain that I was raised on, had never tasted the poverty of a northern mountain village. I thought she would never be able to stand it, never be able to become one with my kinsfolk, work alongside them and share their joys and sorrows. I told her I would go first, see how things were and write to her.

'When I left, my wife packed my food for the journey and bade me farewell light-heartedly, a smile on her lips.

'Back home, I laboured throughout the daylight hours and in the evenings threw myself on the kang to gain strength for the morrow. Weeks and months went by and I never wrote to my wife. To tell the truth, I never thought of her except for a few minutes each night, just before sleep came to me.

'Then she wrote to me. A short letter, written not by a scribe, but in her own hand even though she had had little schooling and knew few characters. But she chose the characters with such care that my soul was seared with their bitterness. She said I had changed my heart and no longer loved her. Why had I not criticized her if she had done wrong? Why had I been afraid to tell her that I was leaving her? Was that how an Armyman behaved?

'I burned with shame and that very day I set out for Hunan to bring my wife back. At a southern station I bought a bottle of oil made with the fiery red chilis that the people of Hunan love to eat and I gave it to my wife telling her that in the mountains we had no oil and that she would find it hard. She gave the bottle of oil to a passer-by, saying that if we had no oil then she would eat none and would not find it hard.

'She never uttered a word of complaint and became one of our best workers. We have four children but she finds time for everything. Last year she was elected Chairman of the Women's Federation. She is an activist in study, in production, in hygiene, in birth-control, in everything that benefits the people.'

He shovelled the food into his mouth to make up for the time he had lost in speaking.

We went back to see his wife and he brought her grain and vegetables and fed her tenderly, wiping the spittle from her lips when she coughed.

The swelling in the neck was larger and the whistling noise when she breathed was louder, showing that the injured structures deep in the neck were still bleeding internally and that the blood was pressing on the windpipe. It was becoming urgent to apply traction in order to steady the injured part and arrest the bleeding.

The young doctor beckoned me outside, clearly dissatisfied with the way things were going. Hesitantly, not wishing to offend me, he told me what was in his mind. 'Ever since you said that she must be transferred to a proper hospital, I have had the feeling that this would not be the right thing to do. It would cost a great deal of money and the journey over bumpy roads might make her worse.

'Did you notice her husband's reaction to your suggestion? His first thought was that to send her to Peking would be a blow to his brigade. That's not because he's indifferent to his wife. I happen to know, from what his mate told me, that the relationship between them is exceptionally warm and close. It's because he, like his wife, is heart and soul devoted to the collective of which they form a part. 'After all, we are supposed to bring modern medicine to the villages, to serve the peasants in the fullest sense of the word, not just to transfer our difficult problems to the towns. Isn't there any other way?'

With an effort, I suppressed a feeling of irritation. I was tired, he was my pupil and twenty years my junior. But his earnestness forced me to reconsider the advice I had given and the more I thought it over, the clearer it became that my advice had been routine and superficial, that I had considered only the medical and not the social aspects of the problem.

As far as the X-ray was concerned, although it would be useful to have one, one could not say that it was absolutely essential. It would not give us any information which was vital for correct treatment and which we could not get by careful clinical examination. If we could do without an X-ray, the only remaining reason to transfer her was in order to apply skull traction.

We went back to look at her again and as soon as I saw her prominent cheek bones, I recalled an alternative method of applying traction. Why not pull on the cheek bones? After all, they are part of the upper jaw which itself is part of the skull. Traction on them must be transmitted through the neck and must have the same effect on the injured part as orthodox skull traction. The cheek bone is a bony arch bridging over a muscle which moves the lower jaw. A hook passed round its lower border would be capable of exerting strong traction. Excited, I asked my colleague's opinion and he enthusiastically agreed.

We decided to make hooks by bending steel wire to the right shape. I stood by the bedside, measured the probable dimensions of the hooks, conjured up a mental picture of the deep anatomy of her face, bent the wire and sharpened the points with a file. We needed a strut to keep the traction cords away from the sides of the face. 'Chopsticks,' exclaimed my colleague and he ran off to the kitchen to get them. They were just the right length, a trifle longer than the maximum width of the face.

We needed a pulley for the cord to run over; the nurse produced a cotton reel. She also brought us bricks to use as weights and went off to sterilize the hooks and to prepare syringes for the injection of a local anaesthetic.

When we explained our plan to the patient and her husband, he didn't seem to understand at first and then he lunged forward and clutched my hand. 'You mean you can treat my wife here? You won't send her away to Peking?' I nodded. He stared for several seconds and then burst into uncontrollable sobbing, his Adam's apple jerking convulsively in his lean, scraggy neck.

There were still many unknowns. We did not know if we would be able to pass the hooks under the cheek bones. We did not know if she would be able to tolerate them. Above all, we did not know if her spinal cord would recover.

I cleaned the skin with alcohol, injected the local anaesthetic, thrust the point of the hook through the skin below the cheek bone and manipulated it until I could feel it pass round the lower edge of the bony arch. Then I pushed it upward and it locked securely in position. Elated, I gave the other hook to my colleague who did the same.

Soon the weight of two bricks was exerting continuous traction on her injured neck. The tense muscles relaxed, the pain went and for the first time since the injury, she smiled and lay at ease, physically and mentally.

We gave her a sedative and explained to her husband, who insisted on nursing her, that every two hours throughout the night he must gently roll her from side to side to relieve pressure on the buttocks and prevent bedsores.

First thing in the morning we went to see the patient and found her still comfortable and relaxed. Her husband had washed her face and combed her hair and clumsily, but with great tenderness, was trying to brush her teeth. His face was wreathed in smiles. 'She is recovering, doctor. Look!' He threw back the bedclothes and she moved the toes of one foot up and down. 'She can also move a finger and she knows when I touch her.' Excitedly he demonstrated all the signs pointing to recovery.

Two days later we had to move to another Commune further to the north. It was already clear that she would make a good recovery for both legs had regained nearly normal power and although one arm was still weak, it too was starting to recover. Many months later, she sent me a photograph showing that in fact she made an excellent recovery and resumed her full activities.

Shortly before we left, a peasant from the patient's brigade arrived with a wad of money. 'Take it back, comrade,' the husband said. 'Take it back and thank them. We shan't need it now. my wife won't need to go to the great city. In this age, the great city comes to us farming folk.'

15

How Fragrant Lotus became a mother

Nobody in the village had ever expected Fragrant Lotus to get married, still less to have a baby, for she was a dwarf, a little over four feet tall.

As for Old Han he had never married, for in the old days he couldn't afford to. Wives had been scarce in these parts because so many girl babies were done away with at birth and there was keen competition for the few girls available. His father had been beaten to death by the Japanese and for most of his childhood and youth, Han had been a beggar. He was not particularly prepossessing, had never had a day's schooling and was never in a position to afford even the meanest dowry. So the years went by and Han expected to remain a bachelor for the rest of his days.

But after Liberation life improved year by year, Old Han threw away his begging bowl, farmed the half acre given to him during the Land Reform, joined in turn the mutual aid team, the Co-op and finally the People's Commune and now ate his fill every day and gradually acquired such luxuries as a quilt, an alarm clock and a Thermos flask. He had money in the bank and was even thinking of buying one of those new transistor radios they were producing in Peking. He had everything he wanted—except a wife.

He was forty years of age, was already starting to wheeze when he climbed the hills, and all the marriageable girls were married. Regretfully he resigned himself to a solitary and childless old age. After all, he pondered, he was lucky to be alive for he was the only one of his family to have survived the man-eating society of the past.

One day he found himself working alongside Fragrant Lotus in the turnip field. She might have been there for hours for all he knew, for he never noticed her until he squatted on the ground for a rest and a pipe of tobacco. Despite the cold air, he was sweating and it was restful to watch her working away with a curiously purposeful, unrelenting rhythm. Ungainly, and yet, in a way, graceful. What a tiny, ugly little dwarf she was! Where did she get her strength and staying power?

Soon he felt chilly and, his pipe empty, he resumed work. Conscious now of Fragrant Lotus, he could hear her humming as she worked, not tunefully, but in a low, melodious voice. What had she to be so happy about?

When the whistle blew for the rest break, they all gathered in the shelter of the cluster of poplar trees and some children came from the village with an urn of hot drinking water and a wicker platter piled high with yellow, conical pieces of steamed corn bread.

Not quite by accident, Old Han found himself sitting beside Fragrant Lotus. The children recited passages from the works of Chairman Mao and the peasants carefully unwrapped their little red books of quotations and joined in. Neither Fragrant Lotus nor Old Han could read but Fragrant Lotus evidently knew them by heart for she recited loudly and earnestly, not mechanically like some of them, but as though she had thought over and valued every word.

'Why don't you join in?' she asked Old Han. 'I don't know the words,' he replied. 'I can't read and no one has ever taught me.' 'You mean, you've never learnt,' she rejoined, in Han's opinion, somewhat reprovingly. And then, more gently, 'Would you like me to teach you?' Old Han grunted non-committally.

Then the children sang songs and Fragrant Lotus joined in, swaying from side to side and clapping her hands to the rhythm. Old Han thought she looked a bit ridiculous and for some reason, felt a little embarrassed. After the rest break he moved over to another part of the field.

A few days later the team held an evening meeting to discuss the knotty question of private plots of land.

During the hard years, the word had come down from somewhere, no one quite knew from where, that the way to increase production was to enlarge private plots and extend the scope for private enterprise. It was argued that this would give the peasants more incentive and as a result, they would work harder. The poorer peasants were not easily convinced. They said they had always worked hard anyway, and that it was not until China had become socialist that they had lived decent, secure lives. The difficulties were only temporary, the droughts and floods could not recur indefinitely and surely the solution was not to weaken but to strengthen the socialist system. But somebody high up had said 'Black or white, a cat that catches rats is a good cat,' meaning that 'isms' didn't matter, that all that counted was how much grain was reaped each year and that capitalism, feudalism or socialism would make no difference to that. The former landlords and rich peasants, with their large families and well-situated houses, thought that was a very clever thing to say and they had enthusiastically cultivated their enlarged private plots, raised pigs and chickens and sold the produce for high prices.

Now this policy was coming under heavy fire and being revealed as part of a plot to turn China back towards capitalism. The hard years had been left behind. The irrigation works of the Great Leap Forward were showing results and year by year the yield of the land was increasing. The Commune had never been so stable and flourishing. The Cultural Revolution was revealing the existence of a faction inside the Communist Party, headed by Liu Shao-chi, which was assiduously working for a restoration of capitalism and which had issued the call to increase private plots and private trading.

Which road did the peasants want to take, the socialist or the capitalist road? That was the essence of the argument about private plots.

Fragrant Lotus, who had never before been known to speak at a public meeting, jumped to her feet and delivered an impassioned speech.

'Look at me!' she said, looking grotesque in the flickering oil lamp. 'I'm a dwarf and until we set up our Commune, I'd never known a day's happiness. I was lucky my mother didn't smother me at birth like she did my younger sisters. In the old society, I could put up with the pain and hunger. What I couldn't stand was the contempt and sneers of the gentry. The landlord used to bring his Sunday guests out to the fields to laugh at me and I could have killed them all. After my mother died I was all alone in the world. Someone suggested that I should join a circus but I would rather have died than do that.

'Now I am happy every minute of the day. I have a huge family. You are all members of my family and I of yours.' Her gesture embraced all the peasants squatting in the shadows. 'I eat my fill, I learn the thinking of Chairman Mao, I sing songs in his praise and I work to build our country and our Commune into a bastion of socialism. All this is because we took the socialist road! Let us do away with private plots entirely and give all our strength to the collective!'

Many peasants murmured approval but some of the older ones were silent. They wanted to think it over. They agreed with reducing private plots but doing away with them altogether was a different matter. After all, in the old society, it had been the ambition of every poor peasant to possess his own plot of land, no matter how tiny it was. Of course, things were different now. Now, collectively, the peasants owned all the land and that was good. But still . . . there was something very comforting, very secure in having a bit of land of one's own, land on which there was no mortgage, no rent. They wanted to think it over. . . .

Old Han had been surprised by Fragrant Lotus's speech. He had been surprised that she had the nerve to speak up in front of all these people. And he had been still more surprised that she was in favour of doing away with private plots. She, like him, had no one to feed but herself and had no need of the full quota of work points and the full grain allocation. She would be better off if she devoted part of her time to her private plot, raising fine vegetables and expensive produce. Yet she didn't do so. . . . He began to feel that there was something very unusual, very admirable about the little dwarf. More and more, without caring whether people noticed it or not he sought her out in the fields and worked beside her.

One day, during the rest break, Fragrant Lotus turned to Old Han and said, 'Old Han, may we study together?' 'Hm—that's an improvement anyway,' he said testily. 'Last time it was "shall I teach you?" All right—let's study together, but you'll find me a poor student.'

That evening they met in the school room and she started to recite 'Serve the People'. . . .

' "Our Communist Party and the Eighth Route and New Fourth Armies led by our Party are battalions of the revolution. These battalions of ours are wholly dedicated to the liberation of the people and work entirely in the people's interests. Comrade Chang Szu-teh was in the ranks of these battalions. . . ." '

'I suppose he was a high-ranking officer,' interjected Old Han.

'No, he was an ordinary soldier who had been given the job of making charcoal when he met his death,' replied Fragrant Lotus.

'Even so, what has it to do with us?' rejoined Old Han. 'We are not in the Communist Party and neither are we in the Army.'

'That's true,' said Fragrant Lotus. 'But in a way, we are both in the "battalions of the revolution" for by our labour and our study we are helping the cause of the revolution. I don't understand it very well myself, but I think it has a lot to do with us. Every time I recite "Serve the People"—even if I only recite it to myself—it makes me feel stronger and more determined. Look what it says—"wholly"—"entirely". Those are big words that express big ideas. New ideas. I feel ashamed that I never had the determination to learn to read. I've had plenty of opportunities during the past four years. If I could read, I could serve the people better than I do.'

Old Han sat silent for a few moments, curiously moved. 'Tell me,' he said, 'how could I serve the people better?'

'Well, you too could learn to read. And you could be more careful in your work,' answered Fragrant Lotus, looking him straight in the face. 'When we were digging up turnips the other day, I noticed that you sliced and damaged many of them.'

'Yes, I didn't care,' admitted Old Han after a pause. 'I felt that they weren't mine and no one would know anyway. I'm glad you told me.'

Through their daily work and daily study, love and mutual respect grew between them and when Old Han asked her if she would marry him, she said, 'Of course I will, Old Han—but I don't know whether I can bear you a child.'

'Whether you can or not, we shall be happy together,' replied Old Han with genuine ardour and indeed marriage seemed to transform him. He shed his dourness and taciturnity, worked meticulously from dawn to dusk and studied in the evenings. He spoke up freely at meetings of the Poor and Lower Middle Peasants Association and he and Fragrant Lotus took the lead in merging their private plots with the collective fields. Within a few months of his marriage, he was elected team leader.

The village peasant doctor was the first person to know when Fragrant Lotus became pregnant. Fragrant Lotus suspected that she might be pregnant but she was by no means sure and she didn't like to say anything to Old Han in case it was a false alarm, for she knew that while he never expected her to have a baby, he would be delighted if she did.

So she asked the young peasant doctor. Although he was young and had only studied medicine for four months during the last slack farming season, he was popular with the villagers and everyone thought well of him. Moreover, his wife had given birth to a baby not so long ago, so he should have gained some first-hand experience.

In fact he turned out to be quite knowledgeable and Fragrant Lotus was glad she had called him in. He examined her carefully and concluded that if she was pregnant, her small size and the narrowness of her pelvis would make it difficult for her to give birth to a full-term child. So he arranged for a consultation with a member of the mobile medical team from Peking.

A few days later Dr Chou visited the village. She had not been long in the countryside and was unaccustomed to travelling long distances on foot. The peasant doctor met her on the outskirts of the straggling village, shouldered her medical bag and, moved by her obvious fatigue, borrowed a donkey, helped her into the wooden saddle and took her to Fragrant Lotus's cottage.

After a brief rest on the kang, Dr Chou examined Fragrant Lotus, measured the width of her pelvis, and told her that she would talk it over with the peasant doctor and let her know their conclusions later on.

When Fragrant Lotus had left the room, she told the peasant doctor that there was no doubt that Fragrant Lotus was pregnant and there was equally no doubt that she couldn't give birth to a full-term baby. The sensible thing to do would be to terminate the pregnancy by abortion. Theoretically there was another possibility. They could wait as long as possible and then try to deliver a live baby by abdominal operation. But having regard to the fact that she was a middle-aged dwarf and that she lived in a remote mountain village, this possibility was hardly worth considering.

The peasant doctor looked dejected. 'Of course, you know the medical aspects much better than I do,' he said, 'but just now when you spoke about facts, you mentioned only some of them. Another fact is that both Fragrant Lotus and Old Han suffered greatly in the old society. Liberation has given them a new lease of life. If they have no child, both their families will die out. I don't know if they will agree to an abortion. Don't you think we should discuss it frankly with both of them before making up our minds? Wouldn't that fit in better with the Chairman's teaching to trust the masses?'

That evening the four of them met in Old Han's cottage. He invited the visitors to sit on the kang and Fragrant Lotus gave them bowls of hot water to drink. As Dr Chou raised the bowl to her lips, she noticed the line of grime around the rim and surreptitiously tried to wipe it off with her finger. Fragrant Lotus noticed it, took the bowl from her, swilled it round, emptied it on the beaten earth floor and refilled it.

'I'm sorry our bowls aren't so clean,' she said. 'It's not easy to wash them thoroughly up here in the mountains for all our water has to be carried on shoulder-poles from a spring in the valley. And brush-wood for boiling the water has to be collected from the mountain-tops.'

Dr Chou smiled apologetically. 'Of course, I understand,' she said. 'It's just my habit to wipe the rim of the bowl. I do it in town as well.'

Her legs were getting numb from squatting on the kang and she shifted her position frequently. Without saying anything, Old Han placed a little stool on the kang for her to sit on.

'How old are you, Fragrant Lotus?' she asked. Fragrant Lotus wrinkled her brow. 'I was born in the year of the Tiger, I think I'm thirty-nine.' The peasant doctor calculated silently. In the Western calendar she would be thirty-eight.

'Anyway, you're getting on to be having your first child,' continued Dr Chou, 'and . . .'

Fragrant Lotus broke in, beaming broadly, 'So I *am* pregnant!' she exclaimed and exchanged triumphant glances with Old Han.

'Yes, you're pregnant,' said Dr Chou, 'but your pelvis is much too small for you to give birth to a baby in the ordinary way. I'm very sorry to have to say so, but we must seriously consider whether the best thing wouldn't be to have an abortion. That would be safe and simple and afterwards we could make sure that you don't become pregnant again.'

When she heard the word 'abortion', Fragrant Lotus folded her work-calloused hands protectively across her abdomen. Tears started in her eyes and she shook her head vehemently.

'What's the alternative to an abortion?' asked Old Han, bristling.

'The only other way is to wait until Fragrant Lotus goes into labour and then deliver the baby through a big cut in the abdomen. That would have to be done in the county hospital.'

'Well, what's wrong with that?' asked Old Han.

Dr Chou chose her words carefully. She didn't want to frighten the couple unnecessarily, neither did she want to bemuse them with big words which they wouldn't understand. But she wanted to make sure that they realized all that was involved.

'Fragrant Lotus is so tiny that I don't think it's possible for her to carry her baby until full term—that is, until it's reached a stage when it's ready to be born. We don't know when she'll go into labour but when she does, the operation must be done very quickly. Delay might be dangerous for the mother and even more dangerous for the baby. How can we quickly get her over the mountains to the county town while she is in labour?'

'I'd carry her,' said Old Han unhesitatingly.

'I know you would,' conceded Dr Chou, 'but she wouldn't find it very comfortable and neither would it be very quick. It might do her harm to be moved so far over rough mountain paths.'

'Couldn't the operation be done here, in our own cottage?' pleaded Fragrant Lotus. 'That would avoid the dangers and difficulties of getting to the county town in a hurry, maybe at night and maybe in bad weather.'

'Of course it couldn't be done here!' replied Dr Chou, glancing round at the earthen floor, the sparse, coarse furniture and the paper-covered windows. 'It's a big operation, not a small one. To do it here, without electric light, without proper equipment, without running water—and without elementary hygiene, would be out of the question.'

Her vehemence brought a momentary silence. Then Old Han, speaking quietly, almost apologetically, asked, 'You're a Communist Party member, aren't you, Dr Chou?' Dr Chou nodded. 'My wife,' continued Old Han, jerking his head towards Fragrant Lotus, 'has told me that members of the Communist Party are wholly dedicated to the people—work entirely in their interests. I believe that's true. But I don't quite understand how you square it with saying that it's out of the question to operate here. It seems to me that to operate here would be in the interests of the brigade, of Fragrant Lotus, and of the baby which we long to have. If I'm wrong, please explain my error.'

Dr Chou was on her mettle now. 'Chairman Mao also tells us that in their every word and every deed, cadres must be responsible to the people. It's a question of responsibility. If anything went wrong, I'd be responsible and I wouldn't feel at ease operating under these conditions.'

At first diffidently, and then with increasing confidence, the peasant doctor expressed his opinion. 'I understand your point of view, Comrade Chou,' he said, using the word 'comrade' to emphasize that he, a member of the Communist Youth League, was talking to a full-fledged Communist Party member who was also his teacher, 'but I don't fully agree with it. We'd all be responsible if anything went wrong, not only you. Of course, you have the responsibility for making the final decision for you have most knowledge and experience. But, morally, we're all equally responsible.

'You say you wouldn't feel at ease operating here and I can understand that, for the conditions here are so different from those you are accustomed to. But ease of mind isn't the main thing. Dr Bethune did bigger operations under worse conditions when there was no choice. Did he have ease of mind? It's true that we have a choice, but if Fragrant Lotus goes into labour unexpectedly, it may be very difficult indeed to get her to the county hospital in time. Couldn't we make such full preparations here that the chances of anything going wrong would be reduced to a minimum?'

Dr Chou thought for a few moments before replying.

'Certainly there's truth in what you say. It's not easy to get out of a rut, to discard deeply ingrained habits and standards. It's all too easy to rationalize things so that one's own interests, such as one's own ease of mind, are made to appear identical with others' interests, when actually they are not.

'Let's sleep on it and decide tomorrow. We must make the right decision and not embark on any rash adventure.'

Next day they met again. This time there was no need for much discussion for they had all arrived at roughly the same conclusions. There would be no abortion. Dr Chou would operate on the kang as soon as possible after Fragrant Lotus went into labour. Old Han would thoroughly clean up the cottage and ensure an adequate supply of fuel and water. The peasant doctor would keep a close watch on Fragrant Lotus and make all arrangements for the operation. As a first step he did blood tests to see whether, in case of need, Old Han's blood could be transfused into Fragrant Lotus, and he beamed broadly when he learnt that his blood was compatible with his wife's.

Fragrant Lotus went into labour in the middle of the night early in the eighth month of pregnancy. The weather was bitterly cold and a gale-force wind was howling through the pines as the peasant doctor hurried to brigade headquarters to telephone Dr Chou. He was glad that it wouldn't be necessary to move Fragrant Lotus on such a night as this.

Then he ran back to the cottage and found that Old Han had piled fuel on the kang stove and was boiling a big cauldron of water. The cottage was spotlessly clean, the window papers had all been replaced and a new reed mat covered the kang. Looking more grotesque than ever with her distended belly, the dwarf was tidying up, lovingly arranging the sheets in the cradle that would soon hold her baby, trimming the wicks in the numerous oil lamps she had borrowed from the neighbours. Whenever she was seized by a labour pain she would momentarily lean against a wall and then, as the pain passed off, full of confidence and happiness, she would resume her preparations.

'Old Han,' said the peasant doctor, 'I think it would be a good idea if I were to take a pint of blood from you in case your wife needs it. It would save time if we had it all ready for transfusion. What do you think?'

'I agree,' said Old Han. 'We said we would do everything to reduce risks to a minimum. I'm ready.'

He lay on the kang, rolled up his sleeve and clenched and unclenched his fist till the veins became prominent. The peasant doctor cleaned the skin with iodine, plunged a needle into a vein and allowed the blood to gush out through a rubber tube into a bottle containing a chemical to prevent clotting.

As dawn was breaking, Dr Chou and the medical team arrived, bringing everything needed for the operation including even a small cylinder of oxygen. She approvingly noted the warmth and cleanliness of the cottage, the bottle of blood standing on the window sill, the cauldron of boiling water and all the other signs of thorough preparation and without pausing to rest, examined Fragrant Lotus and listened to the heartbeat of the child within her womb. 'Everything's fine,' she said. 'Let's start.'

Spinal anaesthesia was to be used so Fragrant Lotus moved to the edge of the kang, rolled on to her side and bent her back as much as she could. At the exact point in the middle of the back, a long, slender needle of special design was thrust deep between the segments of the spine until it reached the tough membrane guarding the spinal cord. This membrane gave a feeling of elastic resistance to the needle and a further carefully controlled push carried the needle point through it into the watery fluid surrounding the spinal cord. After allowing a few drops of fluid to run out, a syringe was attached to the needle and a measured quantity of anaesthetic solution was slowly injected through it. Then the patient was turned on to her back and the lower part of the body was raised so that the solution would remain around the lower part of the spinal cord controlling the legs and abdomen, and would not flow upwards towards the brain.

After a few minutes, her legs started to feel numb and then the numbness spread up her thighs and abdomen as far as the lower chest. When she could no longer feel pain, the abdomen was painted with iodine, sterile sheets were draped over the patient and the surgeon and her assistant, wearing sterile gowns and gloves, began the operation. Dr Chou stood beside the kang while the assistant squatted on the kang on the other side of the patient. The peasant doctor kept a check on the pulse and blood pressure and shone a torch into the wound. Dr Chou operated swiftly and with precision. A few deft strokes with the knife opened the abdomen and exposed the womb. Small blood vessels which had been divided in the course of cutting through the abdominal wall, were grasped in special forceps and tied with surgical silk. The movements of the child could be seen inside the womb.

Now came the crucial stage of the operation.

When the lower part of the front of the womb was incised in order to gain access to its interior and deliver the baby, an unexpected and dangerous snag was encountered. Usually the placenta or after-birth is attached to the middle part of the womb, but in this case it was attached to the lower part, overlapping the line of the incision. To reach the interior of the womb it would be necessary to cut through the after-birth with its many large blood vessels and two dangers would arise. One was haemorrhage from the vascular after-birth and the other was asphyxia of the infant. This emergency called for quick decisions and close co-operation.

'You'd better start transfusing the bottle of blood you've prepared,' Dr Chou told the peasant doctor without looking up. 'She might need it in a hurry.'

The peasant doctor attached tubing and needle to the bottle of blood and crouching on the kang next to the assistant, thrust the needle into a vein in Fragrant Lotus's arm. Soon the blood was dripping into her veins.

The incision in the womb was rapidly deepened until it had gone through the whole thickness of the placenta. The bag of fluid containing the baby was opened, and with a firm but gentle movement, Dr Chou delivered the tiny slippery baby, still attached by its umbilical cord. Within seconds she had tied and severed the umbilical cord and placed the baby on a warm sheet.

While Dr Chou concentrated on the baby, her assistant dealt with the severed placenta from which blood gushed at an alarming rate. She squeezed

160

the cut edges between her fingers but, even as she did so, the peasant doctor reported that the blood pressure was falling and the pulse rate rising—signs of impending shock. 'Give the blood faster,' said Dr Chou. He unscrewed the clamp on the rubber tubing until the blood was running at full speed and gave Fragrant Lotus an injection of Ephedrine.

The assistant quickly separated the placenta and brought the haemorrhage under control. She then injected Pituitrin, which had been prepared before the operation for just such an emergency as this, into the wall of the soft, flabby womb. Immediately the muscle of the womb contracted into a firm, pale, ball of flesh and bleeding from it almost ceased.

Unheard sighs of relief. The peasant doctor checked the blood pressure and found that it had risen to a safe level.

Meanwhile Dr Chou was fighting for the flickering life of the new-born babe which was hardly breathing and whose waxen pallor indicated a dangerous lack of oxygen.

She inserted a rubber tune into the infant's throat and applied suction to remove anything that might be obstructing respiration. Still the baby did not breathe. Without hesitation she removed her mask, took a deep breath, placed her lips over the infant's mouth and nose and gently breathed out. The tiny chest filled with air. After this had been repeated a few times, a trace of colour appeared in the infant's cheeks and it gave a faint gasp—the first sign of spontaneous breathing.

'Quick—the oxygen,' said Dr Chou. The peasant doctor had already attached a face mask to the cylinder of oxygen, and as he unscrewed the valve, oxygen hissed out. Dr Chou held the mask in front of the baby's face. It gasped again. Then a third time and gradually the breathing became regular. Three pairs of eyes were riveted on the baby and after minutes that seemed hours, it gave its first, uncertain cry.

Soon the issue was beyond doubt; the baby was out of danger.

The peasant doctor felt weak and trembling. His voice sounded strange in his ears as he murmured his relief.

Fragrant Lotus lay comfortably on the kang, propped up by pillows, a firm bandage round her abdomen, her cheeks a healthy pink, looking a picture of contentment and happiness.

While the doctors were clearing up and packing the instruments into their medical bags, Old Han was pottering about in the kitchen from which smells of food and wisps of smoke drifted into the room.

Suddenly everyone was ravenously hungry and when Old Han brought in bowls of steaming millet, they fell on it like wolves, munching in silence, pausing only to reach out with their chopsticks for pickled vegetables, fragrant wild mushrooms and fiery red peppers. After the millet, he gave them sweet potatoes, baked on the kang stove, blistered and charred in patches as sweet potatoes should be. Then thin millet gruel with a little fresh cabbage in it, a treat indeed in the depth of winter in the mountains.

'But why don't you give anything to your wife?' asked Dr Chou. 'She must be hungry too.'

Old Han grinned sheepishly, muttered something inaudible and continued to potter around in the kitchen. In due course he came in with a dish of sweet glutinous millet pancakes, fried in oil, garnished with strips of pork, which he placed beside his wife.

Big eyed and incredulous, she looked from the dish to her husband and back again. She had never eaten such food in her life.

'Eat it,' he said in a gruffly tender voice. 'That's what nursing mothers always eat. It gives them strength and helps them feed the baby. . . .'

Happily Fragrant Lotus munched the pancakes. Like the other married women, she had become a mother and was content.

16

Ox tale

It is by no means uncommon for members of the mobile medical teams to give roadside consultations in the course of tramping from village to village, since peasants with minor complaints often prefer to wait for the doctor by the roadside rather than spend time returning home from the fields.

If roadside medical examination is impracticable, it is completely in order to use the nearest cottage for these country folk are very hospitable and open-hearted and take it for granted that a sick man and his doctor have the right to use anybody's cottage. I have given manipulative treatment for slipped discs to complete strangers in the homes of equally complete strangers who happened to live nearby. There is a lot to be said for the innate courtesy and lack of formality encountered in the Chinese countryside.

Here, I want to tell not of a roadside examination of a human patient, but of the riverside examination and treatment of an ox, for mobile team members must learn to be versatile and many-sided.

We had just finished our rounds in a beautiful little village at the top of a steep valley. Our last patient had been the ploughman who a few weeks before had developed a strangulated hernia and, but for a prompt and correct diagnosis by the village peasant doctor, would probably have died. As it was, a team turned out in the middle of the night and successfully operated on him in his own cottage. We had just checked up to ensure that the hernia was cured and had given him permission to do light work.

'Light work!' he snorted. 'The autumn harvest is in and all the work from now until the spring sowing is heavy work. We have to plough the land, spread fertilizer, dig ditches, level terraces and such like. And our ox, doctor, seems to be heading for the stew pot. Please come and see him. You fixed me up and you might be able to cure him too.'

Without waiting for a reply he led the way to a field still strewn with the debris of harvested maize, along one side of which a stony little stream splashed and sparkled in the autumn sunshine.

'There he is. See how thin he is, how his back sags, how rheumy his eyes are.' He pointed to a forlorn looking ox standing in the stream.

'He's hardly eaten anything since it happened. He won't last long at this rate.'

'Since what happened?' we asked. 'Tell us the whole story from the beginning—we don't speak ox language so we can't ask him ourselves.'

He seemed a little put out by our facetiousness, but continued. 'Well, about three weeks ago, we harnessed our two oxen and a donkey to a cart-load of turnips which we were sending to town. There must have been easily two tons of turnips on that cart and since there were a few rivers to cross, we put both our precious oxen on to the job. Of course, the donkey doesn't have much pulling power, but he's useful for setting the pace. He's out in front on a long trace, and without him the oxen would never make the journey before nightfall.

'Well, they hadn't covered more than two li before one of the oxen lowered his head, got his horns under the belly of the other and gave him a jab which would have done credit to one of those fighting bulls I hear they rear in the West. Of course, I don't know if they really rear fighting bulls. In these days with artificial insemination finding its way even into a tiny village like ours, I cannot imagine why people should want to rear so many bulls. They're useless for ploughing or pulling and they eat enormously.'

He rambled on extolling the virtues of oxen and condemning the wickedness of bulls until we guided him back to his story. 'I've no idea what made him do such a thing. Those two oxen were the same age and they'd pulled together over many a long mile. Never a cross look between them. Never a sign of temper. Then, for no reason at all, the one goes and nearly kills the other. Of course, there must have been a reason, but we have no way of knowing it.

'Anyway, this one grunts, lies down between the shafts, rolls up his eyes and sweats like a mule. We had to unharness him and lead him back, leaving the turnips to be collected by a lorry from the county town.

'Next day he developed a big lump on the side of the belly. You can see it from here. There are gurgling noises inside the lump and sometimes it gets bigger and sometimes smaller. If you ask me, he's got the same sort of thing that I had before you operated on me—but not as bad as mine for I would never have lived through the night without that operation.'

We examined the ox and there was no doubt that the ploughman's diagnosis was correct. The ox was suffering from a traumatic hernia of the abdominal wall. The force of the blow had torn a hole in the muscles and fascia of the abdominal wall, and loops of intestine had come out through the hole and were lying coiled up beneath the intact hide. It was a serious condition which would get worse without treatment. We told the ploughman to call in the village vet and he said that he had already done so.

'He agrees that it needs an operation but he says he can't do it. He's never done that sort of operation, doesn't have the instruments, doesn't know how to do it.'

'Sorry,' we said, 'we're in the same position as the vet. No experience. No instruments for ox surgery.'

Perhaps we had spoken too light-heartedly as though it were a matter for joking, for this time the ploughman was annoyed and made no attempt to hide it. 'It's easy for you to talk like that. But I don't think you know what an ox means to a farmer in a hilly place like this. I've seen you medicos round these parts for nearly a year and I know that you help with the harvesting, digging and such like. That's good. The old 'uns like myself remember the time when any lad who'd been lucky enough to get a few years' schooling and who'd learnt how to use the brush and ink block would never soil his hands with the earth that grows his food. He'd grow his fingernails an inch long, wear long sleeves and leech on to some landlord or magistrate so that he could sit on the backs of us common folk.

'You're not like that, but that doesn't mean that you know everything about life in the villages. You just told me to do light work. What I call light work would be very heavy work for you, and what you call light work wouldn't be considered work at all round here. You can joke about not having ox

164

instruments, but if the ox doesn't pull the plough next spring, then we shall have to pull it ourselves. Believe me, that's not light work! We feed that ox all through the year to get two months' ploughing out of him.

'When I was a lad in the prime of my strength, I hired myself out to a landlord on a yearly basis. He wasn't too keen on hiring me at first since I was a bit skinny and he said the skinny ones were the biggest eaters. So I told him I was as strong as an ox. "Strong as an ox, are you?" he said. "We'll see." And he harnessed me to the plough alongside an ox and drove the plough himself. Every time the ox outpulled me and the plough slanted through the earth, that old devil would crack his whip across my shoulders, roar with laughter and shout out, "Come on, you self-styled ox! You're just a heap of ox dung!" '

The ploughman fell silent, offended by our apparent unconcern and lost in recollections of a bitter past. We, for our part, felt deflated. We apologized for our flippancy and promised to come back after we had discussed the problem.

As we walked home, we talked over the events of the afternoon. . . .

'We put his back up by behaving like arrogant intellectuals. We felt that because we had cured his strangulated hernia, he should be eternally grateful to us and laugh at our silly jokes about not having ox instruments and not speaking ox language. There's nothing so wonderful about operating on his hernia. That's what we've been trained to do, trained for many years at the expense of people like the ploughman. We think it's wonderful because it was we who did it.'

'That's right,' another rejoined. 'We overestimate ourselves and underestimate others. We think that peasants merely use their muscles and don't use their brains. But just look how that ploughman diagnosed the ox's hernia and knew that in some ways it was similar to his own. He's had no education but he introduced artificial insemination into this village.

'And look at the scientific achievements of the peasants round here! Look how ingeniously they lead water up the mountain sides to irrigate the high terraces. Look how they have worked out a method for transplanting maize plants from maize nurseries so as to be able to reap two crops a year in spite of the short growing season. Look at our peasant doctors! They've only had four months' medical training, most of them started with only a primary school education and they spend nearly all their time working in the fields. But they are sensible and conscientious and they already do useful work. Just think back. We studied for six years in primary school, six years in middle school and six years in medical college. Eighteen years altogether! And what did we know when we first qualified? I honestly don't think we were as capable of independent work as these peasant doctors. That's because we didn't combine theory with practice. For years and years we poured so-called facts into our brains but, because we didn't use them, they mostly evaporated as fast as we poured them in. Our peasant doctors haven't learnt so many facts, but what they learn, they apply immediately.'

The first speaker intervened a trifle impatiently. 'We've talked enough about what we did wrong. Maybe we were a bit tactless, but that ploughman is too touchy. It's more important to discuss whether we can cure the ox.'

Another member of the team disagreed. 'I'm not so sure that it's more important to discuss whether we can cure the ox than to discuss where we went wrong. Our attitude to the ploughman was wrong and we should learn the lessons from it. It's not just that we were tactless.

'We've all read Chairman Mao's article in memory of Dr Norman Bethune. Mao praised Bethune's sense of responsibility and warmheartedness and said that all Communists should learn from him. He said: "There are not a few people who are irresponsible in their work, preferring the light and shirking the heavy, passing the burdensome tasks on to others and choosing the easy ones for themselves. . . . When they make some small contribution, they swell with pride. . . ."[1] Aren't we a bit like that? Didn't we preen ourselves on our success with the ploughman's operation? Didn't we try to pass on the difficult task of curing the ox's hernia to the vet? Didn't we adopt an irresponsible attitude towards the ploughman's request? Can we say that we showed "great warmheartedness"?'

For a time we fell silent, pondering over the immensely complicated problem of changing one's thinking in a changing world. We thought of Bethune, lean and gaunt, impatient of carelessness, affronted by apathy, burning with an unquenchable inner fire, driving himself and driving others, wholly devoted to the cause of the revolution.

After supper, we made detailed plans for operating on the ox, for it was abundantly clear that we should have to do so.

To make the incision we decided to use the kind of kitchen chopper which is used in every Chinese home for slicing meat and vegetables and for making noodles. It can be sharpened to a keen edge and its weight and strength make it more suitable than an ordinary surgical scalpel for cutting through ox hide.

To stitch the wound we would use the kind of bodkin which the Chinese use for making cloth shoes. To hold the wound open, we would use long-handled bamboo back-scratchers.

Anaesthesia presented a big problem. If the ox would stand still for long enough and if we could find a hollow needle sufficiently strong to penetrate its hide without bending, we could give it an intravenous injection of a strong sedative; but it seemed unlikely that we could meet either of these conditions. A more reliable, albeit cruder, method would be to tie the ox's feet and get a heavy man to sit on its head. If necessary, perhaps we could also administer a sedative by mouth.

As for dressing the wound after the operation, it was ridiculous to think of encircling the ox's vast girth with bandage for, apart from not having enough bandage, we would not be able to apply it while the animal was lying on its side. We decided to stick the dressing in place with rubber solution from a bicycle puncture repair outfit.

When we arrived to perform the operation we found the ox, thinner and droopier than ever, standing in its accustomed place with its forefeet in the little stream. The ploughman approached it from behind and in a trice had its head in a gunny bag. Then he led it to the bank of the stream, threw it on to its side with a quick, skilful movement, and sat on its head while its feet

[1] 'In Memory of Norman Bethune,' Mao Tse-tung, 21 December 1939. *Selected Works, Vol. II, p.* 337.

were tied together and fastened to a post. A bevy of children appeared from nowhere and arranged themselves in rows to watch the performance.

The surgeon sat astride the ox and tried to inject local anaesthetic around the bulging hernia. The needle bent until it looked like a fishing hook. The children tittered. The gunny bag was removed from the ox's head, its upper lip pulled back to reveal the toothless bovine upper jaw and a wad of cattle feed containing a stiff dose of sedative was inserted into its mouth. The ox rolled its eyes, belched, shifted the wad from side to side as though in preparation for swallowing it and then ejected it unchanged on to the ploughman's foot. The children tittered again.

We decided not to bother about an anaesthetic and the surgeon grasped the kitchen knife and made a neat incision around the bulge in the beast's flank. The ox appeared not to feel it and nonchalantly urinated against the surgeon's leg. The titter from the children was audible across the gully.

The assistant held the wound open with back-scratchers and the surgeon dissected out the sac of the hernia, pushed the intestines back inside the abdominal cavity and stitched up the hole in the abdominal wall, layer by layer, overlapping for extra strength. The operation was completed in less than an hour. The children murmured approvingly and went home.

When the rubber solution sticking the dressing in place was dry, the ploughman got off the ox's head, untied its feet and the ox, somewhat unsteadily, made its way to the stream for a drink.

We couldn't think of any appropriate post-operative instructions and so we left the ox in the safe hands of the ploughman and started for home, uncertain whether our operation would prove successful or not.

Three weeks later we went to remove the stitches. The ploughman, full of smiles, told us that the ox was doing well, eating normally and filling out. It was grazing on scrub grass half way up a steep slope, its back straighter and its hide glossier than before the operation.

Unconcerned, as if it were an everyday matter, the surgeon ripped off the dressing. The ox responded with a nimble, well-aimed kick which sent him sprawling. The ploughman observed that it was a pity the children were not present and suggested that it would be as well to hobble the ox. When he had done so, we removed the stitches and were delighted to find that the incision had healed well and that the hernia appeared to be completely cured.

The ploughman, in jubilant mood, saw us off to the edge of the village.

'What days we live in!' he mused. 'We who hungered all our lives, now eat our fill. We were as ignorant as oxen but now the Chairman tells us to concern ourselves with State affairs. We were as separate as grains of sand but now are united solid like a rock. We always drifted aimlessly at the mercy of the wind and tide but now we have a chart and a helmsman. And, to cap it all, the Chairman sends us fine doctors like yourselves who first save the ploughman and then save the ox. I'm sorry if I spoke roughly the other day. Come and see us in the spring and I'll teach you how to plough.'

'We'll come,' said the surgeon. 'You've taught us a lot already and we want to learn more.'

17
No such thing as doom

Granny was starting to feel a bit impatient with her daughter-in-law, who for days had done nothing but sit on the kang, offering the baby her full breast, hopefully sticking her nipple into its mouth. Couldn't she see that the baby was doomed? Why did she fight against fate? Why did she not get on with digging its grave?

Granny pottered irritably through the house on her triangular bound feet, spat demonstratively on the earthen floor and went out into the yard. She had work to do even if no one else had. She turned the stalk frame on which tobacco leaves were drying and cut a golden pumpkin into a long strip, like a yellow dragon, reminiscent of the paper dragons which the villagers used to make at New Year's time when she was a girl. . . . Everyone would line up under the dragon according to size, and parade it round the village, making it writhe and coil just like a real dragon. Once her brother had smoked his pipe in the dragon's head and had puffed smoke out of its fearful nostrils. How the girls had screamed!

She draped the pumpkin strip over a wire stretching from the wild pepper tree to the eaves of the house. The autumn sunshine was warm and a breeze blowing down the valley would soon dry it. If pumpkins were well dried they would last all through the winter and provide many a tasty meal when all the sweet potatoes were eaten and there were only pickled vegetables to eat with the millet.

Then she turned the gourds so that they would dry evenly all over. They were too tough to eat but were well shaped and free from cracks. In a few days she would slice them in half, remove the interiors and dry the shells. She could make at least four good ladles out of those gourds and they would last till long after she was dead and gone. She had made gourd ladles when she first came here as a new bride, so many years ago, while the Emperor was still on the throne. She had oiled and polished them until they turned a rich deep brown and only in the last few years had they started to crack.

She half filled her basket with wild peppers from the heavily-laden tree, and squatted on a stone to remove the shiny, black, oil-rich kernels. Later she would sell both the flesh and the kernels in the Commune supply and marketing station. It would take her a full day to go there and back but she would sell some walnuts too and with the cash would buy paraffin, matches and salt.

She went back into the house, added some brushwood to the kang stove in the central kitchen and rejoined her daughter-in-law who was still helplessly wiping away tiny beads of sweat from her baby's forehead. Granny did not like to show her irritation for her daughter-in-law was a good girl and a hard worker and it was backward for mothers-in-law to abuse their daughters-in-law as they had done in the old days. She spread the peppers and pepper kernels on the kang, squatted next to her daughter-in-law and, as though to console her for the coming death of her child, started talking about her own early married life. 'My first baby was a girl and that was bad, for I had to smother it with my own hands and, believe me, it wasn't easy. I felt towards it just the same as you feel towards that poor little mite who will be dead and buried before the week is out; just the same as all mothers feel towards their first-born. But in those days we were starving and had no way out. Some of us had to die and if a girl grew up she would leave home to get married as soon as she was able to do a little work, otherwise the landlord's running dog would soon be on the scene and, before you knew what had happened, she would be a plaything for the landlord or the landlord's son or both.

'When the Japanese were here things were even worse. They burned down all the outlying villages and drove us into places which they called "strategic villages". They said it was to protect us from the Communists and bandits up in the hills but we'd have been better off without such protection! We couldn't cultivate our land, all our draft animals were commandeered by the Japanese and we had to live on whatever leaves and wild grass we could gather while collecting firewood for the Japanese. Ai-ya-a! I could speak for a month without stopping about the bitterness of those days; the beatings, the hunger, the anger of seeing our local gentry hobnobbing with the Japanese devils, feasting them at our expense, supplying them with our daughters.'

She hawked angrily, her dull old eyes lighting up with hatred and contempt.

The baby suddenly screamed in pain and a jet of dark brown vomit shot across the kang. The pain passed off and the baby slumped into its mother's arms, deathly pale, covered with sweat. The mother, distraught, pressed her child to her bosom, seeking to give it her warmth, her strength.

Steps sounded outside, a hoe was leaned against the wall and the child's father came in. He saw the pain on his wife's face and the ominous streak of dark brown vomit. 'How is she, Ma? Will she live or die?' He spoke to his mother, averting his eyes from his wife.

'She'll die within a day or two. You'd better start digging the grave. Any day now the ground will freeze and then it won't be so easy to dig the grave.'

'Are you sure she'll die? Is there nothing we can do?'

'Of course she'll die. She's doomed. Just smell that vomit. Just see how white she is! It's Fate and it's no use fighting against Fate. In the old days we might have called in the Wise Old Woman. . . .' Irresistibly Granny was drawn back to recollections of her youth. 'I remember the Wise Old Woman in our village. Filthy dirty she was, covered with lice and her hair hanging all over her face. In she'd come waving her horse's tail, singing songs in a queer high voice and speaking words that no one could understand. She'd usually tell us to kill a dog or a chicken and sprinkle its blood over whoever was dying. Of course, we couldn't do so, because if we'd had any chickens or dogs we'd have eaten them or sold them long before. Anyhow, it made no difference. Whether we called in the Wise Old Woman or not, whoever was doomed to die, died. Just like that poor little baby girl of yours will die.

'There aren't any more Wise Old Women in these parts. The last one fell ill and although she treated herself with magic words and potions, she got steadily worse. When she looked like dying, she called in a famous Wise Old Woman from the next village who took the case very seriously and even sprinkled her with badger's blood, which is just about the most powerful remedy there is. But it did no good at all. Just when we were getting ready for her funeral, a travelling traditional doctor came to the village, riding a mule and laden with all kinds of herbs. He used to come this way once or twice a year and although his medicines were expensive, they were very good. He insisted on seeing the Wise Old Woman because he saw it as a contest in skills and he made a powerful dose for her. The Wise Old Woman sneered at him but she swallowed the medicine and within a few days, she started to recover. By the end of the month she was as fit as a flea so she admitted her defeat, burned her magic books and her horse's tail, had her funeral clothes made up into ordinary working clothes, gave up her profession and became an ordinary hard-working peasant. Since then there have been no Wise Old Women in these parts so there is nothing you can do.'

The man shuffled his feet awkwardly. For some minutes he could not bring himself to look at his wife and then he looked up gruffly and said, 'I know what we can do. I'll ask Old Guo's boy to come over and take a look at her. He's a real bright lad—studied in the village school for nearly four years and can read and write hundreds of characters. He was working alongside me today and in the rest-breaks he was telling me about how he's learning to be what they call a peasant doctor. Last year, after the autumn harvest was in and the land had been ploughed, he went off to Four Seas where he studied until the spring sowing. That gave him a full four months and it's amazing what he learnt. He knows how the body works, why it gets ill, how to kill germs and worms and such like. This year he'll go back again to learn some more. When the doctors from Four Seas come this way, he always walks round with them and they tell him what he did right and what he did wrong.

'I'll go and ask him to try his hand on our little 'un. It can do no harm, can it, Ma?'

'No, it can do no harm. She's doomed one way or the other. Let the lad have a bit of practice.'

The mother lifted her eyes pleadingly. 'Call him quickly. My baby is not doomed. I don't believe anyone is doomed.'

The man hurried out of the house, anxious to avoid conflict between his wife and his mother. Of course his mother was what they call conservative but she had a lot of commonsense and was often right.

He clambered over the stone wall his mother had built to keep their pig in their yard. Most villagers didn't mind if their pigs wandered at will, but his mother said that the pig would lose weight clambering all over the place, and if it spent its days visiting its friends, who would get the manure? So she had built a low stone wall and the pig had not yet found a way to climb over it.

The man had been working since dawn and was hungry. He hurried along to Old Guo's cottage and found the family squatting on the kang, eating millet porridge with lumps of sweet potato in it, just like everyone else in the village. Old Guo's wife got a bowl and chopsticks and urged him to join them. They squeezed up to make room for him around the kang table but he wouldn't eat. When he told them why he had come, little Guo jumped down from the kang, grabbed his medical bag, and with an unmistakable touch of pride said, 'Let's go.' 'Finish your dinner first,' said the man. 'A few minutes won't make any difference.' 'I've finished,' said the youth, and showed his empty bowl.

Old Guo watched them go with a smile of satisfaction.

'You see, mother,' he said to his wife, 'our son is a doctor now, a peasant and a doctor. Both. I don't know how much he understands about sickness but he will learn more and, since the patients are all our own folk, he will surely do everything he can to help them.'

Little Guo questioned the mother about her baby's illness and this immediately lowered him in Granny's eyes, for traditional doctors didn't make things easy for themselves by asking questions. They first felt the pulse, for a long time, on both sides, and then they told you what was wrong and you just filled in details when necessary.

But the lad was being taught chiefly in the modern school so it wasn't his fault. The mother answered his questions clearly enough. The baby had been normal at birth and for the first few days had thrived. But gradually its belly had swelled and the bowel movements stopped. Then it started getting attacks of pain in the belly which in the last few days had been accompanied by vomiting. Today the vomit had been brown and stinking and the baby was so weak that it could no longer suck her breast.

Little Guo rummaged in his medical bag and took out a thermometer and a stethoscope. While he was taking the temperature his calloused fingers felt the feeble, thready pulse. The temperature was below normal. He looked at the drum-tight belly and saw the intestines forming an ever-changing pattern as though there were a writhing serpent inside. Suddenly the serpentine pattern became more prominent and the child screamed in pain. The peasant doctor listened to the belly through his stethoscope and heard a cascade of noises, as though fluid were trying to force its way through a narrow outlet. He felt the child's eyeballs and found them to be softer than normal. He pinched up a fold of skin and after he released it, it remained wrinkled and loose like the skin of an old man.

He had learnt about these things last year and he knew their significance. The weak pulse, the soft eyeballs, the wrinkled, old-man's skin meant that the baby was dehydrated; that there was a lack of water in the body. The distended belly, the paroxysms of pain, the vomiting, the sinister coiling up of the intestines, all pointed to intestinal obstruction. He did not know the cause of the obstruction, but he was sure that the stinking vomit and the extreme weakness were danger signals and that unless the obstruction were relieved soon, the child would die. An operation was necessary and only the mobile medical team could perform it.

Little Guo was aflame with excitement. His brigade had trusted him, had sent him to study last year and was sending him again this year. They had given him a splendid leather medical box complete with drugs, syringes and such like. Now was his chance to repay their trust.

He told the mother what he thought, dashed out of the house and raced to the telephone in the brigade headquarters. It seemed ages before he heard Dr Chen's familiar, reassuring voice at the other end of the telephone: 'Yes— of course we can come. We'll come as soon as we can but we must first sterilize everything and the walk will take us at least six hours. It will be dark before we arrive. You must prepare everything so that we don't waste time. Clean up the room, warm the kang, protect the baby from the cold air. If you can inject some saline under the baby's skin it may be absorbed and help overcome the dehydration and make the operation safer. We'll leave as soon as possible and we'll travel fast.'

He ran back to the house and told them the good news. Some real doctors were on the way! He must get ready.

He seized a broom and started sweeping. Granny snorted cynically but she set about replacing the torn squares of paper covering the window. The father brought in a pile of firewood and built up the kang stove.

Little Guo took a syringe and needle out of his medical box, and placed them in the wicker-work bread steamer standing on the cauldron of boiling water on the kang stove. When they were sterilized, he injected saline under the loose skin of the baby's armpits until they were bulging with fluid. He had made what preparations he could and now he could only wait.

In Four Seas village, too, preparations had been completed and Dr Chen and Nurse Douan were ready to leave. Dr Chen had been in the countryside for nearly a year; he knew all the mountain paths, could cover long distances, climb high mountains, cross rivers and was a self-reliant, dependable member of the team. Nurse Douan, young and enthusiastic, was still fresh from Peking, and had not yet toughened herself. She had been one of the first to volunteer to work in the rural areas, was delighted when she was selected and was determined to do well. She never admitted fatigue after a day's tramping over the mountains and never complained about the food, even though it was obvious that she missed the delicacies to which she was accustomed in Peking. She said she liked the dry millet, sweet potatoes and garlic knobs but she ate much less than the others and took a longer time over it.

The remaining members of the team saw them off to the edge of the village.

In high spirits, at a good pace, they tramped along the broad valley beside the fast flowing river. Soon they would have to cross a log bridge resting uncertainly on piles of stones bound together with twisted maize stalks. The logs moved with every step. Some were high, some low; some curved upwards, some downwards; some were thick, some so thin that they seemed certain to break under the weight of your body. They were spaced far apart and a false step or an unexpected gust of wind would send you hurtling down into the torrent below. The first time Nurse Douan had crossed it, she had been terrified and had crossed at a snail's pace, clinging to colleagues in front and behind. This time she was determined to manage alone, for Dr Chen was carrying the equipment on which the baby's life depended and she preferred to take a ducking herself rather than risk pulling him off the bridge.

When they came to the bridge, Nurse Douan said that she would cross first. She removed her cloth shoes, thrust them into her pockets and was about to venture barefoot onto the logs when Dr Chen called out that an old peasant woman was crossing from the other side. They waited while she negotiated the flimsy structure on her tiny bound feet and when she had crossed, she gave the girl a warm reassuring smile. Emboldened, Nurse Douan set off and soon reached the far bank. Her heart fluttering, she squatted on a stone, mopping her forehead, flushed with relief and a sense of victory. She waved to Dr Chen who, sure-footed, soon joined her. Grinning, he patted her shoulder and using a famous analogy by Chairman Mao, he told her, 'You see—the bridge is only a paper tiger! It looks terrible but actually it's not. After a few crossings you trip across like a veteran.'

Their path now left the valley and started climbing into the mountains, becoming ever narrower and stonier as the valley receded into the distance. The sun was getting low and brought out the full beauty of the autumn tints. The bright orange leaves of the apricot trees shone with an intensity which contrasted strangely with their peculiarly black, ungainly boughs. The air was fragrant with the kind of wild lavender used by traditional doctors for moxibustion. Untidy looking briar bushes with clusters of black berries grew across the path.

By now they were sweating but they had no time to rest. At the top of the mountain, the air was cold and dank, and fingers of mist probed down the mountainside and coiled up in the hollows. They hurried downwards.

Down in the valley there were more streams to cross but neither slippery stepping stones nor even single log bridges could deter the girl. They crossed the valley and started to climb the final mountain range which lay between them and their destination. As they climbed, with the sun starting to dip behind the mountains, an eagle attacked a little bird in the bowl of blue sky overhead and Douan clutched Chen's arm as it swooped, talons outstretched. The little bird, sensing danger, dropped out of reach at the last moment and beating the air with panicky wings, flew bravely towards the setting sun. The eagle circled leisurely, gained height and dived again. The end could not be long delayed and at the third attack the eagle seized its prey. Nurse Douan gave a little cry of pity and hurried onwards, her fatigue and fears forgotten, towards the baby in the cottage beyond the mountain.

When they reached the top of the range the sun had set and Douan used her torch. A blister on her foot made every step painful. As they were crossing a stream, she slipped, her cloth shoe filled with icy water and was carried away by the torrent. Desperately she flashed the torch downstream but the shoe was black and there was no hope of finding it. There were now less than three miles to go and the only thing to do was to press on. The sharp stones cut her foot and slowed her down. She urged Dr Chen to go on without her but he said that she would not find her way alone. He wrenched the peak off his cap and tied it round Douan's foot with a bandage so that they could make faster progress. At the entrance to the village they were met by Little Guo who had seen their torchlight in the distance. A few minutes later they were in the warm room, mellow with the light of the oil lamp and hospitable with human smells. Douan sank on to the kang, weary beyond description. Granny brought her warm water to wash her feet and urged her to rest.

Even by the light of the oil lamp they could see that the baby was in a desperate condition. Its breathing was rapid and shallow, its nostrils dilated with every breath and its skin was deathly pale. Very little of the saline had been absorbed from the armpits for the blood circulation was too weak. The pulse could hardly be felt. The child was in a state of severe circulatory collapse and an intravenous infusion of saline was urgently needed. To do this in a tiny baby it is necessary to expose a vein in the arm, dissect it free from the surrounding tissues, insert a fine metal tube into it and tie the tube in place. If the vein is large and the lighting is good, this is not difficult, but under the

173

existing conditions, and with a tiny, collapsed vein, it presented considerable difficulty. They worked fast but with extreme care, and soon the saline was dripping into the vein, replenishing the depleted circulation and bringing a little colour back to the waxen cheeks. The operation could now begin and Nurse Douan scrubbed her hands, donned gown, mask and gloves and arranged the instruments on the kang table, draped with sterile towels. Dr Chen added a sedative drug to the saline in the bottle, prepared other syringes with stimulants and told Little Guo what they were and how to administer them. Nurse Douan squatted on the kang beside the baby so that she could hand Dr Chen the instruments and assist him. Little Guo looked after the intravenous drip and lit up the operation field with his electric torch.

Dr Chen injected local anaesthetic into the abdominal wall and when it had taken effect, he made an incision. Distended coils of intestine immediately extruded through the incision for the intra-abdominal pressure was high. Inserting two fingers into the abdominal cavity, he traced the distended coils of intestine downward until he came to the site of the obstruction. He found that the cause of the obstruction was congenital narrowing of the lower part of the small intestine and that the partial obstruction had become complete when distension produced kinking of the narrowed segment. He straightened out the kink and immediately the fluid intestinal contents started to force a passage through the narrowed segment. The obstruction had been temporarily overcome but to ensure that it would not recur, it was necessary to short-circuit the zone of narrowing by making an artificial communication between the intestine above and below it. While this was being done the child started to whimper and Little Guo injected some sedative. A few minutes later, the pulse became weaker and the breathing shallower showing that the child was on the verge of shock. Little Guo speeded up the rate of the intravenous infusion and injected Ephedrine, a drug which was first discovered in China more than a thousand years ago and which, under its Chinese name of Ma Huang Su, has been used by traditional Chinese doctors ever since.

The baby responded to treatment and when the danger of shock had passed, Dr Chen completed the operation as quickly as possible, returned the coils of intestine to the abdomen and sewed up the incision.

Soon the child was sucking feebly at its mother's breast. Even Granny, who had remained unconvinced throughout, clucked approvingly and went out to prepare a meal for the guests from across the mountains. But before the food was served, Nurse Douan had fallen asleep on the kang. The exertions of the journey, the warmth of the room and, above all, her enormous relief at the successful outcome of the operation, had acted on her like an opiate and she slept like a child for several hours.

Dr Chen and Nurse Douan lived in the house for three days after the operation and only when it was clear beyond all doubt that the baby was thriving, did they prepare to leave.

Granny made a cloth shoe for Nurse Douan to replace the one she had lost and before they left she said, speaking to no one in particular, 'I was wrong to say that the baby was doomed. In the old days it would have been doomed all right, but nowadays it seems that there is no such thing as doom.'

Postscript

Shortly after I started to write this book the Cultural Revolution began and I found myself in the eye of the greatest political storm of all time.

The Cultural Revolution has often been described as a revolution which touches people to their souls.

At the end of the lane where I live, just by the bus stop, is a derelict brick platform, perhaps the foundation of a long-demolished dwelling. Years ago, two berry-brown, white-bearded old men started to meet there to play chess and soon they were joined by other old men from the neighbourhood. In those days, while they played, they kept an eye on their grandchildren. The toddlers have long since grown up and gone to school, but the chess school seems to have become a permanent institution.

The old men arrive early in the morning carrying little wooden stools, stay until lunch-time and reassemble in mid-afternoon. In winter they huddle close together, shapeless in thick padded clothing, smoking long pipes with tiny brass bowls, crouching over a charcoal burner near the chess board. In summer, they strip to the waist and luxuriate in the heat of the sun.

The players merge with the spectators, for in Chinese chess it seems that the problematics are more important than the result. Passengers alighting at the bus stop sometimes dally, size up the game and offer advice. Occasionally I, too, linger for a while, but, tyro as I am, I never have the temerity to make any suggestions.

Formerly, the talk was always of Kings and Generals, Horses and Pawns. Nothing else seemed to matter for these old men. Now it is different. The chess school is splintering under the impact of the Cultural Revolution. The old men turn up with political pamphlets and newspaper editorials. The other day, one of them brought along a big-character poster which he had written in beautiful old-style calligraphy, replete with classical allusions but with a sharp political content, and read it to the assembled company. More and more I hear them arguing about capitalist-roaders, struggle meetings, Great Alliances and Central Committee directives. The chess pieces are losing their magnetism. Politics is taking command.

A factory worker who lives next door but one, an activist in the Cultural Revolution, told me about her eight year old son. He came home from school one day and criticized his father, also a factory worker, for spending so much time breeding goldfish while all round him the Cultural Revolution was raging. His work mates, too, had criticized him for his indifferent attitude to the Cultural Revolution, but this was the last straw! Irritated beyond endurance, he spanked his son on the bottom.

When the mother came home, she called a family meeting to discuss the rights and wrongs of the situation and to resolve the 'contradictions among the people' as Chairman Mao had taught them. Everyone said his piece and finally the father was convinced that his attitude was wrong. He got rid of the aquarium and on the wall behind where it had stood, he pinned up the Chairman's call: 'Be concerned with affairs of state and carry through the

Cultural Revolution to the end!' The little boy slipped out, went over to the Co-op and soon reappeared with another quotation which he fixed beside his father's: 'Use reasoning, not coercion!' . . .

I travel to and from work on the No. 14 bus which must carry a fairly representative cross-section of the population of Peking, for its route takes it past residential areas, shopping centres, Government and Party offices, colleges, hospitals, factories of many kinds, army barracks and, at the end of its run, on the edge of the city, vegetable and fruit Communes.

This bus journey ensures that my working day starts and finishes with a stiff, but highly palatable, dose of politics. Soon after we set off, the conductress announces that the No. 14 bus is not merely a people's bus, it is also a school for the thought of Mao Tse-tung, an instrument of the Cultural Revolution. She leads us in wishing long life to Chairman Mao and good health to Vice-Chairman Lin Piao; she recites a succession of quotations from the works of Mao; she relays his recent directives concerning the Cultural Revolution; she tells us important news items from the morning's newspapers; she sings the first line of songs of the Cultural Revolution and encourages us to join in; sometimes she asks a passenger, especially an armyman if there is one on the bus, to lead us in singing.

The driver co-operates with her. He gets into neutral gear while she is singing so as to reduce the noise of the engine; he calls out the name of the approaching bus stop; sometimes he, too, leads us in song.

The conductress gets off the bus at each stop to help passengers mount and alight. The passengers hold themselves responsible for the comfort and safety of the old, the young and the sick while they are on the bus. When we are not singing or reciting, we talk of the Cultural Revolution among ourselves or glance at the slogans and Dazibaos[1] that cover the streets of Peking and convert the city into a million-volume, ever-changing political treatise.

It's really a unique sort of bus journey, not so much because we learn things we didn't know before, but because of the atmosphere of unity and involvement which prevails on the bus. We feel that we are comrades, united by our common determination to carry through the Cultural Revolution to the end.

When I leave the bus, I always feel like thanking the conductress but I don't do so, because there is nothing to thank her for. She, like so many millions of others, is just doing what she ought to do; she is responding to the call of our day and age and is adding her slight weight to the locomotive of history. . . .

Examples could be multiplied indefinitely to show how China's millions are involved in the Cultural Revolution; how most people are deeply, passionately involved. Grey-beards and school children, country women with bound feet, workers, students, intellectuals, peasants and soldiers, all argue the issues of the Cultural Revolution, all study its documents, all take sides, all participate, all learn, all are moving nearer to the day when, in Lenin's words, every cook will be able to run the State.

Never before have so many people been aroused so fully over issues of such fundamental importance as those of the Cultural Revolution.

Never before has democracy flowered so luxuriantly among the masses of

[1] Dazibao = Big-Character Poster, one of the main means of communication in the Cultural Revolution.

176

the people; never have ordinary people had such free access to all the media of propaganda and communication; never before has there been such a mighty debate.

Truly the Cultural Revolution touches people to their very souls, and inevitably it has touched my soul too.

The demands of the Revolution, my deepening involvement in it, the ever-increasing necessity for political study and my continuing surgical responsibilities, made heavy inroads on my time and energy. As a result, this book has been written in dribs and drabs and this, together with my own inadequacies, has multiplied its shortcomings and omissions.

One striking omission is that it does not describe the Cultural Revolution.

In reading this book, the reader may have been struck by a number of antitheses.

For example, the chapter 'Scaling the peaks' describes the unrestricted, open-handed allocation of funds, materials and personnel in the treatment of the burned steel worker Chiu Tsai Kang, whereas the peasant woman in 'The soldier's wife' would have had to pay for an ambulance to Peking.

Is there an inconsistency, an injustice here? Does this fit in with China's socialist system?

Undeniably, it is a good thing that Chiu Tsai Kang's life was saved and that, as a result, advanced burns centres were established all over China. But if this type of concentrated effort were to be pushed one-sidedly, at the expense of providing elementary health services for the great majority of the people, the good thing could become a bad thing. If antitheses of this type were to be ignored, left to chance, regarded as nobody's business, then undoubtedly they would become exacerbated. Privileged strata would arise, the achievement of the spectacular would become an end in itself and the desire for fame would supplant service to the people as a driving force in society.

Such antitheses have a political origin and they require a political assessment.

The Cultural Revolution has turned the spotlight on them and placed them on the agenda for solution.

Readers will also have noticed that I have frequently indicated the existence of a clash between two lines in medical matters.

For example, in the attack on diseases such as syphilis and schistosomiasis, there was a clash between those who relied chiefly on the political consciousness and enthusiasm of the mass of the people, and those who attached first importance to experts and technique. In the synthesis of insulin there was a clash between those who dared to aim high, give youth its head and boldly open up new paths, and those who advocated caution and gradual progress in the wake of others. In the orientation of medical services to the countryside there was a clash between those who wholeheartedly wished to implement the policy advocated by Chairman Mao, and those who argued for first developing urban medical services and thereafter, step by step according to the availability —or non-availability—of personnel, supplying the needs of the countryside. In the policy of integrating traditional and modern medicine there was a clash between those who were willing to examine the strong and weak points of both schools with an open mind and had confidence that each had a contribution to make, and those who despised one or other school and favoured a policy of separatism. In medical education, there was a clash between those who stressed the importance of the moral qualities and political outlook of medical students, and those who were only concerned with their medical knowledge; between those who appreciated the value of short-course training for medical auxiliaries in order to serve the people, and those who insisted on orthodox six-year courses for all medical workers; between those who regarded practical work and integration with workers and peasants as an essential part of medical education, and those who regarded it as a waste of time.

Clashes of this type were also to be found in industry, agriculture, military affairs, education, scientific work, literature, drama, State planning—in every sphere of activity in People's China.

Although in individual cases, they may have arisen from differences of opinion as to how to achieve the same end, in their summation they reflected two different and opposed types of political thinking, two opposed political lines.

These two opposed political lines within society found organized expression in every level of the state and Party apparatus, right up to the Political Bureau of the Central Committee. The struggle between them was sometimes muted, sometimes shrill, but it was always present. It developed into a life and death struggle between capitalism and socialism, a struggle for the future of New China.

The Cultural Revolution is a culmination of this struggle for the future of China. In a very real sense, it is also a struggle for the future of mankind.

It is impossible, within the framework of this book to describe one of the most important developments of the twentieth century—a development which is not yet completed and which continues to gain in power and momentum. I would, however, like to state my own attitude to it in unequivocal terms.

For nearly fifty years Mao Tse-tung has led the Chinese revolution with a brilliance which incontrovertibly establishes him as the outstanding genius of our age. I regard the Cultural Revolution as his crowning achievement.

It is most necessary and most timely. Without it, there was a grave danger that the revolution would have been destroyed from within and all the gains lost. With it, China's socialist system has been immeasurably consolidated and her advance, at a tempo which will astonish the world, has been assured.

As Vice-Chairman Lin Piao has put it, the losses of the Cultural Revolution have been tiny; the gains vast.

For the first time in human history it has shown how a State under the dictatorship of the proletariat can advance towards the classless society of the future and resist subversion by newly emerging privileged groups.

Already, even before the predetermined stage of transforming society has been fully reached, the flood of letters and articles pouring into the newspapers, reporting achievements and inventions, suggesting new ways of doing things, making proposals and counter-proposals, shows the immense source of creative energy which has been tapped by the Cultural Revolution.

Medical matters, too, figure in this great discourse. . . .

Tachai, the pace-setting People's Commune in the arid Shansi mountains, describes the medical school which it has established in order to train peasant doctors from among its own members. Students and teachers excavated caves from the loess soil to house both the school and themselves. They made their own furniture and teaching materials. They support themselves by daily participation in farm work and earn enough to provide graduates with stethoscopes, drugs and first-aid boxes.

The teachers come from the county hospital and the commune clinic and unlike in our Four Seas school, the course runs continuously for eighteen months. Students take it in turns to work as interns in the clinic for a month at a time.

The peasants of Yukiang county, Kiangsi province, celebrated the tenth anniversary of Mao's poem, 'Farewell to the God of Plague' which he had written to express his joy at the elimination of schistosomiasis from this heavily endemic area.

In his poem, Mao described the bygone Yukiang county in these lines:

'Choked with weeds and incontinent sick crumbles a thousand hamlets, Abandoned to the devil's song were yet more homes.'

Now these same peasants could report that their 1,200 water-conservancy projects not only provide safe drinking water for all, but irrigate the land so abundantly that this year they sold 15,000 tons of surplus grain to the State; that for years they had been unable to find a single schistosomiasis-carrying snail, that stool tests in every child born since 1958 had been negative; that they had successfully resisted repeated onslaughts by capitalist-roaders and that the entire population studies and applies the works of Chairman Mao.

Peasants from the Red Star Commune, Linsia county, Kansu province wrote about their beloved 'barefoot' doctor, Cheng Yu-lu, who when the Commune clinic was established in 1963, formed its entire staff. His formal medical training had been fragmentary but his determination to serve the people to the best of his ability and to learn in the course of doing so, earned him their love and gratitude. Since 1965 he has covered vast distances to treat 2,864 patients and the clinic has admitted and cured more than 800 serious cases. When no beds were available in the clinic, he took three children seriously ill with toxic dysentery into his own bed, sleeping on the floor beside them for a week while he doctored and nursed them back to health.

The article stressed the importance of service attitude in medical work and described how, during the Cultural Revolution, the peasants had repudiated Liu Shao-chi's anti-socialist policy of ignoring the needs of the peasantry and had secured the services of three additional doctors.

The Loyuan People's Commune, Hupeh province, started a lively controversy by describing the co-operative medical service which it had established. Members pay one yuan (about three shillings) a year, the production teams add ten cents per head and patients pay five cents for treatment, receiving medicine free of charge. Of the twelve medical staff, two draw a salary and the remainder are allocated work points like other Commune functionaries, receiving an additional allowance to cover extra expenses. Ninety-nine per cent of Commune members joined between January and December, 1968. They claim that this system makes for earlier treatment, facilitates preventive work, places medical work under the direct control of the users, speeds the development of a fully socialist medical service and fosters unity between peasants and doctors. Some feared that the doctors would be inundated with work and the funds quickly exhausted. However, the twin clarion call of the Cultural Revolution, 'Combat selfishness; repudiate revisionism', must have found an echo in the hearts of the Loyuan peasants, for they cherish their new-born medical system, have always left a favourable balance in the medical funds and have treated the doctors with great consideration.

For several days the 'People's Daily' devoted most of its front page to readers' letters on the subject of co-operative medicine. Most of them welcomed the idea as fitting in with the existing level of rural development and with Chairman Mao's directive that in medical work, the stress should be on the countryside. Some favoured a relatively higher contribution from collective funds and a lower one from Commune members. Others advocated that the service should be free at the time of use and still others proposed a differential between chronic and acute sickness.

The Tanwang production brigade in Shensi province described how for ten years it had been running a maternity home entirely on its own resources. More than 5,000 babies had been delivered without tetanus of the new-born, puerperal fever or any other mishap. There were four midwives, all concurrently farm workers, under the leadership of sixty year old Communist Party member Tang Hsiu-lien who, after attending a midwifery course in 1952, had tirelessly answered calls from her fellow peasants. In 1957 she had been elected delegate to the Third National Conference of Women and had been received by Chairman Mao. One stormy night, while on her way to a woman in labour, she slipped and injured her arms and legs, but she crawled nearly a mile along a muddy track to complete her mission.

She has now trained three other peasant midwives and between them, at trifling cost to the brigade, they run a comprehensive ante-natal and maternity service.

The medical section of the People's Liberation Army has provided many examples of the impetus given to health work by the Cultural Revolution. Perhaps the most inspiring is the successful removal of an enormous abdominal tumour from peasant woman Chang Chiu-chu. Her husband, railway worker Tsui Ping-wu, brought her to the little People's Liberation Army clinic in a horse-drawn cart, his wife kneeling in the cart, propping up her body on her two hands, for she had been unable to lie down for many months. She was pale and haggard and had the apathy of hopelessness.

Her husband gently carried her into the clinic and spoke to the People's Liberation Army men. 'Comrades,' he said, 'I know you are not highly qualified specialists and that this is only a rough and ready clinic. But you are loyal to Chairman Mao and share his class feelings. Please help my poor wife. She has been under sentence of death for four years and you are our last hope.'

He told how four years before she had been admitted to a well-known Peking hospital where a piece of the tumour had been removed for microscopic section and a diagnosis of inoperable retro-peritoneal sarcoma of low malignancy had been made. She was told that since radiotherapy was ineffective, nothing could be done, and was sent home to die. The tumour grew until her hands couldn't meet round her belly and, filling half her chest, made breathing very difficult. She returned to the hospital in Peking but the surgeon used words that neither she nor her husband understood. He showed little interest or humanity and sent her home again.

The People's Liberation Army men saw this as a political rather than a medical challenge; a challenge which they were bound to accept. At a meeting of the Party Committee the head of the clinic, Che Li-yi, said, 'When I joined the People's Liberation Army at the age of thirteen, it was just such a poor peasant woman who led my donkey over the hills to where I could find the armymen. During the bitter years of war, it was just such poor peasant women who made shoes for us, carried stretchers, hid and nursed our wounded, shared our every weal and woe. Chairman Mao led us in fighting for decades precisely in order to liberate such people. Even if there is only one chance in a hundred of saving her life, we must strain every nerve to seize that chance. And if we fail, at least we must ensure that our class sister is comforted by our love for her. It is only counter-revolutionary trash like Liu Shao-chi who don't care a damn for the people. This is not just a question of surgical technique. It is a question of which side are we on.'

The struggle began. The difficult task of healing Comrade Chang's mental wound, dispelling her apathy, restoring her confidence and winning her active co-operation, was given to a young male nurse for no women were attached to this unit. Chang was shy and resented having a young man attend to her intimate toilet. He asked whether they should ask for a female nurse but was told to persevere. He did this so patiently, talked to her so naturally and showed such warm sympathy, that gradually her shyness vanished. Then he spoke to her of politics, of his life in the army, of his family, of the contrast between the old and new, of the Cultural Revolution. He explained that the callous treatment of which she had been a victim was incompatible with socialism and represented something which the Chinese people had been called upon to smash. Her confidence grew and she began to believe in the possibility of cure. She told her husband, 'If I die during the operation, please ask the People's Liberation Army men to carry on and remove the tumour from my body so that they will learn how to cure others after me. But I don't think I'll die.'

Meanwhile the doctors investigated her condition with the greatest possible thoroughness. They re-examined the microscopic section which had been made four years before. With the help of other hospitals they made thirty scientific tests including a complex angiographic examination to reveal the blood supply to the tumour.

They studied Mao's statement that 'Man has constantly to sum up experiences and go on discovering, inventing, creating and advancing. Ideas of stagnation, pessimism, inertia and complacency are all wrong.' And they came to understand that if, at a certain stage in the development of medical science, a particular disease could not be cured, this did not necessarily mean that it was incurable, but that knowledge at that time lagged behind reality.

Their investigation of the case, together with the fact that in four years she had not become seriously emaciated, led them to believe that the tumour was probably benign and that a cure was possible.

181

They prepared for the operation as for a battle. Everybody, including cooks, cleaners, patients and gardeners, went into action. Everybody had something to contribute. They considered every possibility, every conceivable contingency before, during or after, the operation. Their slogan was 'To make a suggestion is to catch an enemy!' They preferred to make 10,000 unnecessary preparations rather than neglect one which might endanger the life of the patient. Out of innumerable proposals there emerged 120 concrete measures which were summarized under ten headings. Three different types of anaesthetic apparatus were assembled but still the team responsible for anaesthesia were not fully satisfied. At the last moment they improvised a fourth apparatus which in the event, proved to be the most satisfactory.

At 7.30 a.m. on 23 March 1968, confident and relaxed, Chang Chiu-chu lay on the operating table. After nearly ten hours of meticulous surgery, during which 7,520 ccs of blood were transfused, the base of the tumour was revealed and two huge blood vessels were seen to be closely adherent to it. The decisive point had been reached. Unhurriedly, Che Li-yi, armyman since the age of thirteen, proceeded to separate the adhesions and ligate the blood vessels.

In tense silence the operation was completed and at 7.30 p.m. a tumour, weighing 45 kilogrammes (99 lbs) was removed.

Microscopic examination showed that it was in fact benign.

The stitches from the 95 cm. long incision were removed on the sixth day, and two days later she got out of bed.

By September, she was helping to gather an abundant wheat harvest, a living testimony to the power of the forces released by the Cultural Revolution.

I was one of half a million people who visited an exhibition where the tumour was on display and where the full epic story could be heard in minute detail.

There were lessons of great import to be learned on that visit. . . .

Notwithstanding record-breaking industrial and agricultural output and such feats as completion of the mighty bridge across the Yangste river at Nanking well ahead of schedule, the gains of the Cultural Revolution have been so far mostly in the field of politics. These provide the basis and the driving force for the material advances which surely will change the face of China in the coming months and years.

It is difficult to write about the Cultural Revolution without running into a plethora of superlatives. This is not merely because it is gargantuan in its dimensions. Even more, it is because it is so new in its concept, so bold in its execution and so ambitious in its objectives. It sets itself no less a task than discovering how Man can make the leap from the past millenia of class society to the Communist society of the future. It has many facets. It has uncovered, routed, and thoroughly discredited the anti-socialist faction within the Communist Party headed by Liu Shao-chi.

It is an unprecedented movement to disinfect society, to clear away all pests, to expose political degenerates, backsliders, careerists, no matter how high their positions; to prise out the spies, renegades, traitors, all those whom the Chinese so graphically describe as 'Demons and Monsters'.

It is a vast demolition operation to bring down the age-encrusted edifice of institutions, customs, values and morals of the man-eating past, to clear away the rubble and to drive the foundation piles for the society of the future.

It is tempering China's youth, inheritors of the gains so dearly won by their forebears, the generation on whose 'softness' the imperialists rely to bring about a peaceful reversion to capitalism, in arduous and complex class struggles.

It is a movement to equip the seven hundred million Chinese people with the most advanced, scientific knowledge of the laws of development of society, with Marxism-Leninism in its most developed form, the teaching of Mao Tse-tung.

It is an exploration to discover forms of organization and of government which will be proof against corrosion by bureaucracy and nepotism.

It is the most stringent testing, the most rigorous rectification of the Chinese Communist Party in its nearly fifty years of existence.

It is all these and much more.

History may see it as the harbinger of the emergence of Communist Man; as the fanfare proclaiming the entry of the future on to the stage of the present.

In this book I have described some of New China's achievements in the field of medicine. Similar or greater advances have been made in every other field, and especially in the most important field of all—the revolutionization of the political standpoint and moral qualities of the Chinese people.

I am confident that as a result of the Cultural Revolution, the achievements of the coming decades will dwarf those which I have had the privilege to witness.

At some future time, when it becomes possible to see things in clearer perspective, to present a more or less all-round, balanced picture, it may be that I will sketch those facets of the Cultural Revolution of which I have had first-hand experience.

But the huge task of evaluating and describing the Cultural Revolution, as a whole, will be done by abler pens than mine.

Wounds

Norman Bethune

This remarkable document was written by Dr Norman Bethune shortly before his death from blood poisoning, contracted while operating on a wounded Chinese soldier.

The kerosene lamp overhead makes a steady buzzing sound like an incandescent hive of bees. Mud walls. Mud floor. Mud bed. White paper windows. Smell of blood and chloroform. Cold. Three o'clock in the morning, 1 December, North China, near Lin Chu, with the Eighth Route Army.

Men with wounds.

Wounds like little dried pools, caked with black-brown earth; wounds with torn edges frilled with black gangrene; neat wounds, concealing beneath the abscess in their depths, burrowing into and around the great firm muscles like a dammed-back river, running around and between the muscles like a hot stream; wounds, expanding outward, decaying orchids or crushed carnations, terrible flowers of flesh; wounds from which the dark blood is spewed out in clots, mixed with the ominous gas bubbles, floating on the fresh flood of the still-continuing secondary haemorrhage.

Old filthy bandages stuck to the skin with blood-glue. Careful. Better moisten first. Through the thigh. Pick the leg up. Why it's like a big, loose, red stocking. What kind of stocking? A Christmas stocking. Where's that fine, strong rod of bone now? In a dozen pieces. Pick them out with your fingers; white as dog's teeth, sharp and jagged. Now feel. Any more left? Yes, here. All? Yes. No. Here's another piece. Is this muscle dead? Pinch it. Yes, it's dead. Cut it out. How can that heal? How can those muscles, once so strong, now so torn, so devastated, so ruined, resume their proud tension? Pull, relax. Pull, relax. What fun it was! Now that is finished. Now that's done. Now we are destroyed. Now what will we do with ourselves?

Next. What an infant! Seventeen. Shot through the belly. Chloroform. Ready? Gas rushes out of the opened peritoneal cavity. Odour of faeces. Pink coils of distended intestine. Four perforations. Close them. Purse string suture. Sponge out the pelvis. Tube. Three tubes. Hard to close. Keep him warm. How? Dip those bricks into hot water.

Gangrene is a cunning, creeping fellow. Is this one alive? Yes, he lives. Technically speaking, he is alive. Give him saline intravenously. Perhaps the innumerable, tiny cells of his body will remember. They may remember the hot, salty sea, their ancestral home, their first food. With the memory of a million years, they may remember other tides, other oceans and life being born of the sea and sun. It may make them raise their tired little heads, drink deep and struggle back into life again. It may do that.

And this one. Will he run along the road beside his mule at another harvest, with cries of pleasure and happiness? No, that one will never run again. How can you run with one leg? What will he do? Why, he'll sit and watch other boys run. What will he think? He'll think what you and I would think. What's the good of pity? Don't pity him! Pity would diminish his sacrifice. He did this for the defence of China. Help him in your arms. Why, he's as light as a child! Yes, your child, my child.

How beautiful the body is; how perfect its parts; with what precision it moves; how obedient; proud and strong. How terrible when torn. The little flame of life sinks lower and lower, and, with a flicker, goes out. It goes out like a candle goes out. Quietly and gently. It makes its protest at extinction, then submits. It has its say, then is silent.

Any more? Four Japanese prisoners. Bring them in. In this community of pain, there are no enemies. Cut away that blood-stained uniform. Stop that haemorrhage. Lay them beside the others. Why, they're alike as brothers! Are these soldiers professional man-killers? No, these are amateurs-in-arms. Workerman's hands. These are workers-in-uniform.

No more. Six o'clock in the morning. God, it's cold in this room. Open the door. Over the distant, dark-blue mountains, a pale, faint line of light appears in the East. In an hour the sun will be up. To bed and sleep.

But sleep will not come. What is the cause of this cruelty, this stupidity? A million workmen come from Japan to kill or mutilate a million Chinese workmen. Why should the Japanese worker attack his brother worker, who is forced merely to defend himself. Will the Japanese worker benefit by the death of the Chinese? No, how can he gain? Then, in God's name, who will gain? Who is responsible for sending these Japanese workmen on this murderous mission? Who will profit from it? How was it possible to persuade the Japanese workman to attack the Chinese workman—his brother in poverty; his companion in misery?

Is it possible that a few rich men, a small class of men, have persuaded a million poor men to attack, and attempt to destroy, another million men as poor as they? So that the rich may be richer still? Terrible thought! How did they persuade these poor men to come to China? By telling them the truth? No, they would never have come if they had known the truth. Did they dare to tell these workmen that the rich only wanted cheaper raw materials, more markets and more profit? No, they told them that this brutal war was 'the Destiny of the Race', it was for the 'Glory of the Emperor', it was for the 'Honour of the State', it was for their 'King and Country'.

False. False as Hell!

The agents of a criminal war of aggression, such as this, must be looked for like the agents of other crimes, such as murder, among those who are likely to benefit from those crimes. Will the eighty million workers of Japan, the poor farmers, the unemployed industrial workers—will they gain? In the entire history of Wars of Aggression, from the Conquest of Mexico by Spain, the capture of India by England, the rape of Ethiopia by Italy, have the workers of those 'victorious' countries ever been known to benefit? No, these never benefit by such wars.

Does the Japanese workman benefit by the natural resources of even his own country, by the gold, the silver, the iron, the coal, the oil? Long ago he ceased to possess that natural wealth. It belongs to the rich, the ruling class. The millions who work those mines live in poverty. So how is he likely to benefit by the armed robbery of the gold, silver, iron, coal and oil of China? Will not the rich owners of the one retain for their own profit the wealth of the other? Have they not always done so?

It would seem inescapable that the militarists and the capitalists of Japan are the only class likely to gain by this mass murder, this authorized madness. That sanctified butcher; that ruling class, the true State stands accused.

Are wars of aggression, wars for the conquest of colonies, then just Big Business? Yes, it would seem so, however much the perpetrators of such national crimes seek to hide their true purpose under the banners of high-sounding abstractions and ideals. They make war to capture markets by murder; raw materials by rape. They find it cheaper to steal than to exchange; easier to butcher than to buy. This is the secret of all wars. Profit. Business. Profit. Blood money.

Behind all stands that terrible, implacable God of Business and Blood, whose name is Profit. Money, like an insatiable Moloch, demands its interest, its return, and will stop at nothing, not even the murder of millions, to satisfy its greed. Behind the army stand the militarists. Behind the militarists stand finance capital and the capitalist. Brothers in blood; companions in crime.

What do these enemies of the human race look like? Do they wear on their foreheads a sign so that they may be told, shunned and condemned as criminals? No. On the contrary, they are the respectable ones. They are honoured. They call themselves, and are called, gentlemen. What a travesty of the name! Gentlemen! They are the pillars of the State, of the church, of society. They support private and public charity out of the excess of their wealth. They endow institutions. In their private lives they are kind and considerate. They obey the law, their law, the law of property. But there is one sign by which these gentle gunmen can be told. Threaten a reduction in the profit of their money and the beast in them awakes with a snarl. They become as ruthless as savages, brutal as madmen, remorseless as executioners. Such men as these must perish if the human race is to continue. There can be no permanent peace in the world while they live. Such an organization of human society as permits them to exist must be abolished.

These men make the wounds.

In Memory of Norman Bethune

21 December 1939

Comrade Norman Bethune, a member of the Communist Party of Canada, was around fifty when he was sent by the Communist Parties of Canada and the United States to China; he made light of travelling thousands of miles to help us in our War of Resistance Against Japan. He arrived in Yenan in the spring of last year, went to work in the Wutai Mountains, and to our great sorrow died a martyr at his post. What kind of spirit is this that makes a foreigner selflessly adopt the cause of the Chinese people's liberation as his own? It is the spirit of internationalism, the spirit of communism, from which every Chinese Communist must learn. Leninism teaches that the world revolution can only succeed if the proletariat of the capitalist countries supports the struggle for liberation of the colonial and semi-colonial peoples and if the proletariat of the colonies and semi-colonies supports that of the proletariat of the capitalist countries. Comrade Bethune put this Leninist line into practice. We Chinese Communists must also follow this line in our practice. We must unite with the proletariat of all the capitalist countries, with the proletariat of Japan, Britain, the United States, Germany, Italy and all other capitalist countries, for this is the only way to overthrow imperialism, to liberate our nation and people and to liberate the other nations and peoples of the world. This is our internationalism, the internationalism with which we oppose both narrow nationalism and narrow patriotism.

Comrade Bethune's spirit, his utter devotion to others without any thought of self, was shown in his great sense of responsibility in his work and his great warm-heartedness towards all comrades and the people. Every Communist must learn from him. There are not a few people who are irresponsible in their work, preferring the light and shirking the heavy, passing the burdensome tasks on to others and choosing the easy ones for themselves. At every turn they think of themselves before others. When they make some small contribution, they swell with pride and brag about it for fear that others will not know. They feel no warmth towards comrades and the people but are cold, indifferent and apathetic. In truth such people are not Communists, or at least cannot be counted as devoted Communists. No one who returned from the front failed to express admiration for Bethune whenever his name was mentioned, and none remained unmoved by his spirit. In the Shansi-Chahar-Hopei border area, no soldier or civilian was unmoved who had been treated by Dr Bethune or had seen how he worked. Every Communist must learn this true communist spirit from Comrade Bethune.

Comrade Bethune was a doctor, the art of healing was his profession and he was constantly perfecting his skill, which stood very high in the Eighth Route Army's medical service. His example is an excellent lesson for those people who wish to change their work the moment they see something different

187

and for those who despise technical work as of no consequence or as promising no future.

Comrade Bethune and I met only once. Afterwards he wrote me many letters. But I was busy, and I wrote him only one letter and do not even know if he ever received it. I am deeply grieved over his death. Now we are all commemorating him, which shows how profoundly his spirit inspires everyone. We must all learn the spirit of absolute selflessness from him. With this spirit everyone can be very useful to the people. A man's ability may be great or small, but if he has this spirit, he is already noble-minded and pure, a man of moral integrity and above vulgar interests, a man who is of value to the people.

Mao Tse-tung

Index

189

gastro-enteritis, 132
George III, 83
Germany, 11, 25, 70, 111, 119, 187
goitre, 132
gonorrhoea, 85

haemorrhoids, 12, 75
Haian county, 87
Hailungkiang, 128
Haldane, J. B. S., 11
Harvey, 75
herbalism, 29–30, 79, 124, 170
hernia, strangulated, 163, 165
Hitler, Adolf, 11, 16, 17
Hong Kong, 83
hook-worm, 132
Hopei province, 46, 91, 129
Hsingku county, 87
Hua To, 75
Huai, River, 26
Huang Ti, Emperor, 71
Hulunbu League, 86, 87
Hunan, 73, 149, 150
Hupeh province, 179

impetigo, 145
'In Memory of Norman Bethune'
  see Mao Tse-tung
India, 83, 128, 185
Indonesia, 145
infantile paralysis, 50, 130
Inner Mongolia, 30, 86, 90, 140
Italy, 16–17, 185, 187

Japan, 18, 70, 153, 169
  and anti-Japanese war, 27, 40–1
    48, 76, 134, 185–7
  and 'Manchukuo', 129
  treatment of China, 22, 28, 38,
    83, 107, 149
Jenner, 76
Journal of Traumatology, 110 n. 1

Kansu province, 76, 179
Kiangsi province, 87, 89, 92, 179
Kiangsu province, 87, 88
King, Ambrose, 85 & n. 1
Korea, 126

Kuomintang authorities, 31, 38, 70,
  71, 85, 149
  army of, 27, 66, 83, 86, 97
Kwangtung province, 87

Lai, D. G., 83 n. 1
Lenin, 25, 176
leprosy, 32, 37–8, 75, 92
Lhasa, 36, 37
Lin Piao, 176, 178
Linsia county, 179
Liu Shao-chi, 128, 154, 179, 181, 182
London, 25, 49
  in blitz, 24
  in 1930s, 11, 12, 15, 16

Ma Hai-teh, Dr, 86 n. 1, 87
malaria, 75, 92
malnutrition, 50, 94, 125
Mao Tse-tung, 63, 172
  and Cultural Revolution, 123,
    175, 176, 177, 180
  and 'Farewell to the God of
    Plague', 179
  and 'Foolish Old Man Who
    Removed Mountains, The',
    48, 90 n. 1
  and 'In Memory of Norman
    Bethune', 90 n. 1, 166 & n. 1,
    187–8
  and Marxism-Leninism, 111, 122,
    183
  and memorial meetings, 68
  and 'On Contradiction', 117 n. 1
  and 'On Practice', 114 n. 1
  and 'On the People's Democratic
    Dictatorship', 55 n. 1
  and 'Our Study and the Current
    Situation', 58 & n. 1
  and People's Liberation Army, 38
  and 'Present Situation and Our
    Tasks, The', 97 n. 1
  and 'Problems of Strategy in
    China's Revolutionary War',
    57 n. 1
  and 'Serve the People', 90 n. 1,
    155
  and 'United Front in Cultural
    Work, The', 76 n. 1
  leadership of, 96, 101–2, 113

191

Singapore, 22
Sinkiang, 61
skin grafts, 40, 43, 56, 108–10
slipped discs, 163
smallpox, 75–6, 125, 130
Stalin, Josef, 25
Swatow, 83 n. 1
syphilis, 82–93 *passim*, 177

Taiyuan, 38
tetanus, 125, 180
'Three Old Articles', 90
Tibet, 28, 36, 37, 140
Tientsin, 80
Ts'ao Ts'ao, 75
tuberculosis, 18, 30, 125, 131, 133, 139
typhoid fever, 21, 125, 130
typhus fever, 21, 125, 132

ulcers, 36, 37, 78, 94, 145
'United Front in Cultural Work, The', *see* Mao Tse-tung
US News and World Report, 84 ns. 3 & 4
United States of America, 24, 70, 120

and First Opium War, 83
and Korea, 126
and Kuomintang army, 27, 97
Communist Party in, 187
scientific workers in, 128, 139
syphilis in, 84
treatment of burns in, 107, 110

venereal disease, 18, 82–93 *passim*, 125
Venereal Diseases, 85 n. 1
Vietnam, 84
vitamin deficiency diseases, 18, 125

Wang, Dr, 145
Wardlaw, 115
Whangpoo, River, 23
whooping cough, 125, 130
Winfield, Dr, 126
Wöhler, 111
Wu, Dr L. T., 83
Wutai Mountains, 187

Yangtze, River, 95, 182
Yenan, 68, 107, 144 n. 1, 187
Yukiang county, 179
Yunnan, 140